The WELLNESS JOURNEY

M. VANCE ROMANE

BlueStone

Canadian Cataloguing in Publication Data

Romane, M. Vance, 1949–
   Wellness journey

   Includes idex.
   ISBN 1-896880-02-9

   1. Autogenic training. 2. Romane, M. Vance, 1949– I. Title.
RC499.A8R65 1997   615.8'512   C96-910728-5

Printed in Canada

Edited by Sherry Roberts

𝓑𝓵𝓾𝓮𝓢𝓽𝓸𝓷𝓮 𝓟𝓾𝓫𝓵𝓲𝓼𝓱𝓮𝓻𝓼
23-33293 Bourquin Crescent East, Abbotsford, B.C. V2S 1Y2
(604) 855-6595   Fax (604) 857-9408

Contents

This book is dedicated to my mother who gave me the belief that I could achieve my greatest potential by maximizing the use of the powers of my own mind. When I was a young boy, my mother gave me this single quotation handwritten on a white piece of paper:
"The greatest discovery of my generation is that human beings by changing the inner attitudes of their minds can change the outer aspects of their lives."—William James

Let's Be Friends

I risk a lot writing this book. Often we may help others more by listening than by advising. No two people can agree on everything. I don't expect you to agree with everything in this book. However, please keep an open mind and use what is useful to you in enriching your life. If you don't agree with something, let's agree to disagree and still be friends.

If you allow yourself to do so, you will find that you may become so absorbed with this book that time passes quickly. You may find that many of your worries, fears, and anxieties magically vanish as you read the words in this book. As you become a friend with the brain powers of your inner mind, you will find that many surprise solutions to your difficulties will surface. You also will find that every day you will feel a greater sense of your own individual power of choice, self-control, and empowerment.

Much of this book is based on personal experience—the things I have learned and experienced in my life and in the field of hypnosis. Because I think example is the best teacher, I will share with you events from my life. I'll also share the experiences of some members of my family. I'd like to introduce you to my children.

I most admire my son Vance, 12, for his kindness and caring about other people. Vance is quieter than the girls. He is perceptive and compassionate to other people's needs. He is a whiz on the computer and, if he is not teaching me how to use the computer, he is doing a complicated operation on the computer for my business.

Elizabeth, 13, has a love for animals and currently has a Syrian hamster named Sunshine, who she walks with a leash; a small

Chihuahua dog named Amigo; and a leased appaloosa horse named Shadow. She enthusiastically volunteers for the Society for the Prevention of Cruelty to Animals. Elizabeth is bright as well as being highly perceptive to people's underlying thoughts and motives. She has been a vegetarian since age two, when she asked why the food was bleeding and became disgusted when she learned animals were killed to produce meat. I most admire Elizabeth for her love of our animal friends and her perceptiveness. Elizabeth also has a love for performing in live theater. She dances, sings, and acts.

My oldest child, Diana, is 15. Her main interests are computers and her friends. She has a fine "soulmate" named Jason, who has taught her about computers. I'll never forget when Diana and I visited my psychologist friend, Dr. Ivan Bilash. Diana probably was about two years old and Ivan put a relatively complicated puzzle of wood blocks on the floor to occupy her. Diana instantly placed all the blocks into the proper slots with lightning speed. I was astounded. With all honesty, I could not have solved the puzzle as quickly as she did. A goal-oriented, quick learner and intelligent child, Diana has won numerous awards and educational grants for her school fund-raising activities and superior school grades.

I love all my children dearly. My only regret is that my touring has kept me away from them for 60 to 80 days a year. These regrets have been balanced in part by my passionate desire to serve my fellow Canadians by helping them to be healthier and happier. Fortunately, this work that I have loved so greatly also has helped me to meet the financial needs of my family. In short, it has been satisfying to help people, while at the same time earning a living.

I hope this book helps you. And if it does and you'd like to share your experiences with others, send your ideas to me:

Vance Romane, Box 75177, White Rock, British Columbia, Canada V4A 9N4

Please let me know if I can include your idea in my next book. If your idea does go into my new book, I'll send you an autographed copy as a gift as soon as it is published.

Your friend,
VANCE ROMANE

1

Don't Miss the Journey while Rushing Somewhere Else

According to Statistics Canada (1991), about 20 percent of men will be deceased by age 65. This reminds me of the old song, "Enjoy Yourself, It's Later Than You Think." Fortunately for women, the figure is only 11 percent. Every cigarette, each slice of meat, each spoon of butter, every time we rush from one place to another, each daily stress make our coronary arteries stiffen and resist the flow of blood.

I heard a story about a lady who organized a family get-together with relatives coming from many different cities. However, her sister and her family could not come because her sister's life was "too busy." The sister said that she would come next time. Somehow I cannot help but recall what Virginia Satir once said at a workshop I attended: "We would all be a lot nicer if we were not so busy."

Sadly, the sister who did not attend the family get-together died in an automobile accident and was unable to attend the next family event. The sister who is still alive remains greatly disturbed that they never had that last time together.

Or consider the story of a doctor who was trying to convince two of his friends, who were also doctors, to go on an exotic dream vacation with him. His friends weighed their choices and worried if they could afford to take the time off work, if they could leave their patients in the care of someone else, if the office would continue to run smoothly without them. This reminds me of the often quoted phrase: "No one ever says on their deathbed, I wish I'd put in more hours at work."

Finally, all three doctors decided to go on their planned fantasy trek to South America. When they returned after a month or so, their patients were doing just fine and their offices were running smoothly without them. Shortly thereafter, one of the men died and within a few years, all three had died. None of the men lived to be 60. Because one never knows how long one has on this beautiful and most fascinating planet earth, I always say, enjoy every moment.

Enjoy Every Moment

To enjoy every moment, it helps if you are functioning in mind and body at your very best. I hope that you are in reasonably good health; you love yourself and feel confident; you are loved and you have many good friends; your life is an exploration, a most interesting journey; and you are relatively free of any serious financial worries. I also hope that you are thankful for any gifts life has given to you, for each of us has special talents. Most of us live far better than kings and queens of centuries past.

I also hope that you are relatively free of any major problems. If you have a serious problem such as blindness, or if you are confined to a wheelchair, or even if you have cancer or AIDS, I hope that you have learned to reframe your attitude. Perhaps through rational thinking and mental housecleaning, you can cope or adjust to your life situation in the most positive way possible or even learn a valuable lesson about life from the experience.

If life is not beautiful to you, if you do not treasure every wonderful moment of life, if you have an emotional, spiritual, physical, or even a financial problem, this book is written for you. If you feel a lack of something in your life or if you feel that you have lost a sense of control in your life, then I truly believe that you will benefit immensely from my ideas. You can experience mental cleansing, greater happiness, and a feeling of control over your life. I do not want to take credit for developing all the ideas, for they are centuries old. I have learned them from thousands of others. I would like to share the techniques that I have learned to achieve a feeling of almost constant happiness, peace of mind, and contentment. This is a gift everyone should have.

I was not born with any special skills to achieve this great

2

happiness. If anything, I was born into life with many personal handicaps that I decided to surmount in my early teen-age years. My personal problems challenged me to overcome the unfortunate, to see the best by changing lemons into lemonade.

Over a span of more than three decades, thousands of people have approached me at my seminars with the belief that I am perfect, enlightened, or that I have special inborn powers. However, I *learned* all the wonderful tricks and techniques I know to enjoy a life of almost perfect bliss. When people talk with me personally, they realize that I do not wish that they ascribe to me great mental powers or abilities. Instead, they quickly realize that I support their self-acceptance and self-empowerment.

I think of the prisoners in concentration camps who survived and those who did not. Were the patterns of thinking, such as the degree of their mental strength or "will to survive," of vast importance in keeping many alive? Or, perhaps it was finding meaning in the experience?

How often do we hear of the spouse of a loved one dying and the surviving spouse, now with a huge void in his or her life, losing the "will to live." There are too many reports of husbands and wives dying within a short time period to conclude otherwise. Shock and stress can kill if one does not have a set of beliefs or philosophy that allows one to cope.

How often do we hear of the person who retires to enjoy their "golden years," but quickly thereafter dies. The will to live may dissolve with the termination of work, regular patterns, and many job-related relationships—and death may come prematurely. It is so important to develop interests throughout life that will be enjoyed in the golden years. In fact, I have found that it is far better to focus upon doing things to enjoy living, instead of focusing on thoughts of avoiding sickness and death.

I have truly been fortunate to have a wonderful neighbor named Mary. Mary lives in her own home, alone, at over 91 years of age. Mary lost her husband many years ago. She also lost a son. Her other children and their families live in England and Ontario, Canada. However, Mary lives on, celebrating her birthdays surrounded by her adoring friends in British Columbia. Her positive attitude continues to attract friends who will help her to fulfill any needs she may

3

have. She is a member of a local church and has met many wonderful friends there as well. Friends regularly take her for groceries, to her hair stylist, and to restaurants. They invite her over for home-cooked dinners and, occasionally, they do small repairs in her home.

I find her a pleasure to be with, and we frequently invite her for meals or parties in our home. She never has a complaint. It is a bit of a nuisance to her that her eyes are failing, but not a tragedy. When she outlived her husband and her son, she continued on with her love of people. Her hearing is excellent. Despite a stooped frame and weakened body, she continues to care for a beautiful garden in her large yard. She has help with the lawn, but does much of the gardening herself.

Mary could write a book on her early life with her husband. The two of them traveled the world filming eclipses. Her real life stories and scrapbook of photos could rival the script, exotic locations, and dangers of adventure movies like *Raiders of the Lost Ark.* As we left her 90th birthday party, Mary said: "You have all made this day wonderful for me, and I'll see you on my 100th!"

Control Your Destiny

Successful control of our thoughts is critical for all aspects of our life. If we do not make it our goal to control our own mind, the internal information in our mind and body and the influences of our external environment will control us. We must make a conscious, rational decision to control our destiny. This sense of empowerment will give us better health in mind, body, and spirit. In addition, our inner mind has an endless capacity for creativity and healing. This is the genius within, the 24 hour-a-day workhorse that assists us in our physiological functioning and our everyday life.

Our inner and outer world is a direct reflection of the information we feed into our mind. The sources of information come through all our senses, especially what we see and hear. Whatever we dwell upon—healthy thoughts, neutral thoughts, or unhealthy thoughts—will show up in our life.

If you believe the world is hostile and you are chronically fearful, your body is highly stressed. Spiritual people tend to believe that the world is nurturing, caring, and supportive. By "spiritual," I refer to a positive, optimistic outlook about life.

Herein lies the key. For total happiness and maximum health, it is necessary to tap into the file cabinets of stored information and creative wisdom of the inner mind. This is our gift from the Creator. When I speak of the Creator, it is not my intention to convert agnostics or atheists to a certain religion. Far from it! Instead I say, "Let us together simply look around and see the magnificent stars, the sun, the moon, the sky, the earth, the trees, the oceans, the unlimited variety of trees, flowers, plants, animals, and humans. Then, let us wonder what incredible force, entity, or being has created all this for us to enjoy."

Personal Experiment

Before going to sleep tonight, write down a question such as: "Where is the perfect holiday for me?" Or perhaps, "Should I marry Jennifer?" However, one question per experiment is enough for one evening. Read this over a few times and allow yourself to fall asleep while you are thinking about it. Keep a pencil and paper by your bedside. Your inner subconscious may reveal important information to you in the middle of the night, when you first awaken in the morning, when you are relaxing in a bath or while walking down the street. An intuitive answer may come to you "out of the blue." You can ask the same question several nights for revelations.

Enjoy the Vastness and Wonder of Creation

While imagining the endless outer space, many remain in awe, confused as to the exact beginning of life, the planets, and the solar system. With thoughts of this nature, I am always reminded of William Shakespeare's writings: "There are more things in heaven and earth, Horatio, than are dreamed of in your philosophy."

Consider the magic of our body's own incredible breathing system; our circulatory system, which delivers oxygen and nutrients all over the body; our cardiovascular, gastrointestinal, and immune systems. What a marvelous mystery! Two seeds come together and join like magic. A unique, special, one-of-a-kind human is born. The head, the internal organs, the eyes, ears, nose, mouth, arms, and legs all form from a pre-programmed plan. No two fingerprints are the same. No two voiceprints are the same.

We cut ourselves, and our skin miraculously heals itself. Old cells are replaced by new cells; hair grows; nails grow. We can see, hear, feel, touch, and taste. We can think, create, and invent. We rapidly can change food into skin, blood, bones, hair, and teeth. Our hands and fingers do so much for us. Our legs and our feet take us thousands of miles. I do my best to give thanks every day for all the good that has come to me. I guess that is why I usually enjoy every moment. If I slide off the road to bliss, I encourage and excite myself to get back on track rapidly!

I think it is unfortunate when we forget how amazing we really are. We show respect for the Creator by enjoying and being thankful for all the good in our life. And when we lose this appreciation, it is usually because we have an excess of negative programming from ourselves and/or others. The result is low self-esteem and a feeling of a loss of control over our own life and destiny or just general unhappiness.

The Results of Rushing Through Life

The constant rushing in the life of most people leads to stress; body breakdown; neglect of children; self-abuse with alcohol, drugs, excessive food, and cigarettes; and a dangerous lifestyle. Many unhealthy habits are simply an attempt to escape into a socially acceptable suicide or just an attempt to temporarily numb or escape from our hurting feelings.

Patients come to the "medical magician" for instant help and want the pill, the needle, the operation, or the wave of a sorcerer's wand to make what is undesirable disappear effortlessly and rapidly. If the culturally accepted healer makes the problem vanish, many simultaneously go back to the lifestyle that caused the problem in the first place. At other times, often the real cause of the problem is guilt and a need for punishment, a need to forgive oneself, a need to forgive others, a need to clear negative programming from others as well as negative self-talk. Positive self-talk also may include telling others how well you feel. Your very words may strengthen and reinforce your feelings and condition of health, wealth, and success.

2

How Brain Power Works

Our ability to use our brain power energy is evident in experimental research. For example, if you are asked to test your hand grip strength, you will register as having greater strength if you are first hypnotized and told that you are strong and powerful.

Another experiment is to tell a hypnotized person that his body "is stiff and rigid, as stiff as an iron bar and as strong as steel." Then the rigid body of the hypnotized person is placed between two chairs, with his head on one and his feet on the other chair. A tremendous weight may then be placed upon the body while suspended in mid-air between two chairs. This has been called the body catalepsy test by theatrical hypnotists. Care must be taken not to do this with a person who has back problems. I have seen up to four people stand upon the body of one hypnotized person suspended between two chairs.

I've often said to my seminar audiences: "Who talks to you more than anyone else? You do! And you have to be careful what you repeat over and over to yourself." Sometimes, in response to the question of "Who talks to you more than anyone else, a man will blurt out: "My wife!" Well, if someone does talk to you a lot, I hope that the talk is mostly positive and encouraging.

The Power of Positive Words

Imagine how nice it would be, if from day one, our parents and teachers focused upon positive and encouraging words; imagine what we would learn. Words create pictures in our head. The pictures create the release of chemicals and hormones in our body. The chemicals and hormones create feelings. The feelings create behaviors—positive or negative.

The more senses we use to create positive, vivid 3D mental pictures, then the more powerful will be the electrical and chemical reactions in the body. Visual images are matter. Therefore, in creating these positive mental images, you should use the senses of seeing, hearing, feeling, smelling, and tasting. Add emotion and the effects are even stronger. You can add emotion by having strong motivations or powerful rewards. If what we want is much greater than what we have, an energy may be created to motivate positive action to realize the vision. You can create confidence and emotion by remembering times when you felt successful. Many people do not achieve success, because they are insufficiently motivated.

If a hypnotized person is told that he is in a prize fight, running a race, or that he is being chased by a dangerous animal, his pulse will beat more rapidly because of the imagined experience.

Anyone Can Be Hypnotized

Virtually anyone can be hypnotized. Difficulty hypnotizing arises in clients who are intoxicated, mentally challenged, or who have serious illnesses of the mind. Being hypnotized does require concentration or some degree of cooperative focusing of brain power energies. Children usually are easier to hypnotize than adults. This is because children have excellent imaginations, and they usually are able to relax more easily than adults.

Being hypnotized is quite safe. *However, it is important that only positive suggestions be given to the hypnotized person.* For example, positive suggestions may be given to encourage a person to get proper nutrition, plenty of water, regular exercise, adequate rest, and sufficient sleep.

An automobile used with training and good judgment is safe— and so is hypnosis. Hypnosis is totally safe in trained hands. Hypnotized people should only be told what you want them to do, not what you don't want them to do. A hypnotist should eliminate: "You will not do this or that." Stage entertainers must remember to remove personality changes from the mind of the client before arousal from hypnosis.

Hypnosis is used in medicine to treat arthritis, alcoholism, allergies, asthma, behavioral disorders, burn patients, colitis, coronary disease, drug abuse, epilepsy, hypertension, insomnia, migraine headaches, nail-biting, narcotic addiction, obesity, pain, peptic ulcers, reading disorders, school phobia, skin disorders, stage fright, stuttering, thumb-sucking, warts, and cancer.

Methods of Hypnotism

There are an unlimited number of methods of hypnotism. My favorite is simply asking a person to close her eyes upon hearing each number that I count and to open her eyes in between counts. Hypnosis may be deepened by asking the person to take a few deep breaths while simultaneously saying: "Just allow yourself to go deeper and deeper, relaxing with each breath." Asking the client to imagine a heavy feeling coming over her eyelids will further deepen the hypnosis as she realizes she is really following the suggestions.

The first task in hypnotizing is helping the person to feel comfortable. The client must understand that he will not be asleep, but actually super-aware. His mind will be concentrated, and his body will feel totally relaxed. Feeling comfortable with the hypnotist, the experience, and the room will facilitate hypnosis. A few people take longer to be hypnotized than others, because they have difficulty "letting go." Men and women are equally hypnotizable.

When you are hypnotized, you may not know it. You may feel tingling, heaviness, lightness, floating sensations, watering of the eyes, and eyelid fluttering. Time may seem to pass quickly. Or, you may just feel extremely relaxed with your attention concentrated upon the hypnotist's voice.

You Are Super-aware

You are super-aware. You may hear sounds that you were not aware of in your everyday life. The sense of hearing becomes acute. Yet, you also can become so involved with the hypnotist's words that you temporarily shut out everything around you.

Brain wave tests show that a person is more awake than asleep while he is hypnotized. Just by a simple hypnotic suggestion, you may be made to feel alert, clear headed, and refreshed, upon coming out of hypnosis. Sometimes, people may feel for a short time a little sleepy after hypnosis, if the method of "awakening" was not done correctly.

Animal Hypnotists

Even animals can hypnotize and be hypnotized. Watch how animals use their eyes to fixate attention on each other. Some animals cause their prey to become rigid, while staring at them. Then the animal attacks the "hypnotized" prey. Most so-called "animal hypnosis" involves merely pressing the correct nerves, thus causing body immobility.

A recent news story from Edinburgh told of the world's first canine hypnotist. The dog named Oscar co-stars with a hypnotist named Hugh Cross. When the dog was lost, Cross paid a reward of $7,700 (Canadian) to the finder of his valuable partner. When I was a teenager, my father owned race horses. Horse trainers often asked me to hypnotize race horses to win!

You Can Reject Suggestions

A hypnotized person is always aware that the hypnotist is talking to him, so he can reject suggestions. Hypnotized people are not zombies. Research has proven conclusively that people in hypnosis will not do anything illegal or immoral—unless they would do it anyway, even without hypnosis.

When hypnosis ends, most people remember what happened during hypnosis. Those in deeper levels of hypnosis may have spontaneous amnesia and forget all or part of the experience.

Many people can be hypnotized for the first time instantly, in seconds. Post-hypnotic suggestion is even faster. A person given a post-hypnotic suggestion goes back into hypnosis at a certain cue word, gesture, or upon hearing a certain musical selection; he or she can return to the hypnosis state as quick as the blink of an eye. A scent, taste, or touch also may be used to cue a suggestion. This is truly rapid or instantaneous hypnosis. It can also be indirect, disguised, or subliminal hypnosis. Thousands of stores now broadcast background music with anti-theft messages subliminally embedded into the music.

Subliminal Influence

Can suggestions aimed at our subconscious mind without our conscious awareness result in changes in our behavior? Current research is ambiguous, with support for and against the possibility of such effects. Research does seem to indicate that there is a greater likelihood of success if the person is highly motivated to want the change that is to be generated by the suggestions.

Deepening Hypnosis

You can further deepen the hypnosis by asking the person to imagine a wave of relaxation spreading over his entire body, from the bottom of the feet to the top of the head. You might tell a hypnotized person that his right arm has a balloon attached to the wrist and that the helium gas, lighter than air, is pulling his arm upwards. Then say: "Every time you breathe in, your arm grows lighter and floats higher ... it is bending at the elbow ... the back of the hand is moving toward your face ... as it brushes your face gently, you double your relaxation ... you double your hypnotic state."

These procedures also can be used to deepen self-hypnosis. You could begin by staring at an object and then allowing your eyes to grow heavy and to close. All the while you can be giving yourself mental suggestions that your eyes are growing heavy, that every breath relaxes you deeper, that your body is relaxing from your feet to your head.

Upon reaching a reasonable depth of hypnosis, positive suggestions are fired into the subconscious. Only a light hypnosis state is required for eliminating unhealthy habits. For surgery, a deep state of hypnosis is needed. Deep hypnosis is not as suitable for self-hypnosis. If you go too deeply into a trance while engaged in self-hypnosis, you will lose the ability to give yourself suggestions. You may even drift into an ordinary sleep. Using emotions, the five senses, and imagery—plus repetition—a powerful change in one's life may be experienced. This change may be so rapid that only one session is required. However, further reinforcement is usually needed to ensure permanent success.

Inner Genius: Use It or Lose It

Creating new behavior and actions will bring you health, wealth, and happiness. The patterns of thinking and the skills necessary to achieve success in all areas of mind, body, and spirit healing can be learned. Whether for good mental and physical health or to just put food on the table, these techniques are of unlimited value.

11

Perhaps when a problem or need arises, the question may be: "What should I do that will satisfy my needs, be fulfilling, and be realistically possible?" The real answers lie within our own mind, the subconscious, the inner world. Help is available anywhere, anytime, for free. When we invite, trust, and allow our inner mind to do the work it was designed to do, miracles and magic happen. With practice, this invisible ability is easier to use and it becomes more natural and automatic. With a lack of use, it becomes harder to access. This priceless power is our inner genius.

3

The Connection Between Mind and Body

With absolute certainty, our thoughts can control brain waves; turn on or off the release of certain hormones; control bleeding and clotting, respiration, pulse, the muscular activity of the gastrointestinal system, and even alkalinity and acidity of our body fluids. Current research clearly shows that feelings of hopelessness and helplessness suppress the immune system. Why is it that a wife or husband often dies shortly after the death of a spouse? Is the cause of death heartbreak or a "broken heart"?

The connection between mind and body is being established by research of biochemical and physiological changes related to states of mind. These affect general health and healing from disease. Our state of mind will show itself in our health, our relationships, and our finances.

Our magical body normally attempts to mend itself with preprogrammed input for healing. A lifestyle of unhealthy habits and negative thinking interferes with that normal mending process. Heredity factors aside, there is much we can do to heal ourselves. We have the ability to control many of the things that make us sick, such as stress.

We have long recognized the damage stress can do to the body and to mental and emotional functioning. With stress, a variety of symptoms may occur:

- **EMOTIONAL:** anxiety, worry, frustration, bad temper, nightmares, unhappiness

- **MENTAL:** poor concentration, forgetfulness, confusion or feeling "spaced out," negative attitude, low productivity
- **PHYSICAL:** tension, appetite or weight change, stomach aches, headaches, heart palpitations, teeth grinding, tiredness, insomnia, aching muscles, restlessness, skin rashes (the skin is a mirror to the emotions), constipation, back pain, high blood pressure, cold hands or feet
- **SPIRITUAL:** apathy, loss of purpose, wanting a "magical" cure, unforgiving
- **RELATIONSHIPS:** loss of intimacy and sex drive, lonely, nagging, angry, intolerant, suspicious of others, manipulation of others

Every thought or image creates reactions of a chemical and electrical nature throughout the body. For years, theatrical hypnotists such as Ormond McGill have shown audiences how cutting a lemon in half and then describing the bitter, sour, mouth-puckering taste of the juice can cause the salivary glands of the members of the audience to secrete. Our internal thoughts and imagery create chemicals that communicate to cells, tissues, and organs. If thinking about a yellow, juicy, bitter, sour lemon can cause salivation, what can these stressful events do to our body, mind, and spirit:

- Death of a loved one
- Marriage
- Divorce
- Serious injury or illness to oneself or a close family member
- New employment
- Loss of employment
- Retirement, loss of purpose, boredom
- Pregnancy
- Child leaving home
- Financial woes
- Arguments with spouse, in-laws, or employer
- Changes in habits, residence, school, job
- Vacations with busy airports, car rental line-ups, lost baggage, traffic jams

We all know how thoughts can affect the flow of blood and sexual response. A visualized picture will activate the visual cortex of the brain, but an imagined sound will activate the auditory cortex.

When I tell one person or an audience of thousands to inhale and exhale a few deep breaths, to imagine each part of their body relaxing, to use all their senses and recall a favorite place of peace and tranquillity, the benefits of relaxation are elicited. The breathing slows down and becomes slightly deeper, more regular, smoother. The heart rate slows down.

A relaxed body and mind are far healthier than a stressed body and mind. A relaxed mind possesses inner peace and a feeling of self-control. We have a greater feeling that we can say "yes" and "no" to people and situations in our life. Virginia Satir might have said that at this time in our life we can more easily accept what fits and discard what does not. With this deep relaxation, a profound feeling of euphoria may occur due to the release of natural healing chemicals produced by our body. A trick I have used to remind myself to relax includes placing a small blue dot sticker on the face of my watch, on my wallet, or on my car window.

Again, our thoughts can create heaven or hell for us. This applies to the individual, to a country, and to the world. Imagine a home where all comments are positive and encouraging between husband, wife, and children. Imagine a school where all comments are positive, pleasant, and empowering among the principal, teachers, and students.

Here is a list of proven activities to help you achieve greater peace of mind. (They are adapted from an article I wrote, which was published in *The International Journal For Professional Hypnosis,* Vol. IV, No. l, p. 10-11, 1989.)

A Checklist of Techniques for Combating the Effects of Stress

- Talk to a friend, counselor, minister, or physician.
- Make an appointment for deep muscle massage.
- Use deep breathing exercises. Breathe in a deep breath through your nose all the way down to the diaphragm, the lower part of your body. Babies are more relaxed than adults and breathe more deeply. Adults generally are high chest breathers and need to learn again how to breathe deeply. After inhaling a deep breath through your nose, hold it for a few seconds, then breathe out a long slow breath through your mouth. As you breathe in, imagine that you

are filling up a glass from the bottom to the top and the glass is your body from your waist to your neck. As you breathe out, imagine that you are emptying a glass from the top to the bottom.

- Tense up all parts of your body, one part at a time, for a few seconds each. Then, let go and relax each part of your body. Pause a few seconds after relaxing each part of your body, then go on to tensing and relaxing the next part of your body. You may wish to begin by lifting your shoulders as if you were trying to touch your ears. Hold the tension for about one minute. Be aware of all the sensations, then let go gently and relax. You can repeat this exercise of tensing up the shoulders and letting go several times. You also can do this with other parts of your body. Exercises of tensing up and letting go can be done by tensing and raising your eyebrows high; pressing your lips together; stretching your arms or legs straight and stiff like an iron bar; bending your hand or foot backwards or forwards; holding the breath a few seconds; squeezing the buttocks together, etc. These exercises dissolve tension in the body and relax the mind as well.

- Change your diet to include less salt; less sugar; less alcohol; less fat; less meat; less coffee; and up to eight glasses of water daily, preferably distilled water. Eat plenty of fruits, vegetables, fish, poultry, and whole grain cereals and bread. Follow your physician's advice.

- Be a non-smoker.

- Enjoy relaxing music. Classical and new age music may induce slower, deeper breathing.

- Drive to a peaceful park, forest, beach, mountain, or meadow.

- Exercise with a brisk walk, hike, swim, bicycle. Go to a gym. Buy or rent your own equipment.

- Play a voice cassette for stress reduction or read a relaxing book such as a travel book.

- Read a book about stress reduction. I recommend *You Can Learn to Relax* by Dr. Samuel W. Gutwirth.

- Take a couple of days off and go on a quiet, relaxing vacation.

- Attend a stress reduction class at the local hospital.

- Use self-hypnosis brain power methods: Lie down and relax your body, step by step from the bottom of your feet to the top of your head. Recall or create a peaceful place in your imagination. Use all your senses to make the image as real as possible. Really "be there" to the best of your ability. Enjoy every moment.

- Start a new hobby such as painting, ceramics, sailing, tennis, or yoga.
- Take a self-assertion course at a college or continuing education center.
- Meditate: Sit quietly with your eyes closed. Slowly focus your mind upon one word such as "calm" or "peace" or "relax." Some just choose the word "one." Allow that word or image to roll around in your mind over and over and over. Any word, image, or sound that makes you feel relaxed is fine. When your mind wanders, that is all right. Just refocus on that one word again. If another thought intrudes, let it come and then let it go. If you fight an unwelcome thought, it will strike back harder. In such cases, I may imagine a river, with negative or intruding thoughts flowing away forever, as a piece of driftwood may flow away never to be seen again. At other times I visualize a stone dropping in a quiet lake. I watch a circle forming in the water because of the stone dropping. As the circle disappears, I allow another stone to drop and watch the circle form in the water again and then vanish. This can be most relaxing when repeated over and over.
- Have a warm bath at 92 degrees Fahrenheit, with pleasant bath oil.
- Drink chamomile tea.
- See a foot reflexologist.
- Listen to a comedy recording, audio, video or movie.
- Do several stretching exercises.
- Volunteer to help others for diversion. Engage in new activities; develop new friends. I am not sure where this quotation comes from, but it certainly reinforces my feelings: "It is one of the most beautiful compensations of this life, that no man can sincerely try to help another without helping himself." I know of one patient who felt depressed, as if life was not worth living, yet she forced herself to go out and do volunteer work in a hospital with those far less fortunate than herself. Seeing those living with more serious problems, made her problems seem less important. By helping others, she was able to climb outside of her own world of worries. Her mind became absorbed in a new train of thought, helping someone else to be happy. Another depressed patient who had a

strong religious faith was told to pray for everyone she knew. Soon after, she also was feeling better. Both patients solved their problems in a way that worked for them. However, in both instances, the cure was helping others. Depression frequently is a reaction to a severe loss, often with a guilt feeling connected to the loss. This is best helped by consultation with a clinical psychologist or a psychiatrist.

- Add variety. Make a change in your daily routine, dress, route to work, furniture arrangement, etc. Such changes also are useful for breaking habits such as smoking and overeating. By changing the visual stimuli in your environment, it becomes easier to change the habits.

- Set-up a regular time to relax—take a "relaxation break" instead of a coffee break.

- Change your attitude. Convince yourself that you have a choice as to which reaction you make to every event. Think of someone you know who always seems to remain calm and poised, no matter what happens. Model or emulate their attitudes and behavior.

- Tell yourself you do not always have to be the winner, to be right. When you know someone has upside-down logic and they cannot be reasoned with, it is sometimes useful to say: "You *may* be right." You can *appear* to say that they are right, but you can quietly agree or disagree in your own mind. Most arguments are trivial events anyway. Most of the worries and concerns we have today are forgotten by tomorrow.

- Avoid being a workaholic by over-scheduling or over-committing yourself. Even if your work does give *you* enjoyment, how does it affect the people you live and work with? Make your personal and family life a priority over other demands. If your work causes you excessive stress, listen to your body and make the appropriate changes. Delegate work to others, then trust them to look after it.

- Avoid "keeping up with the Jones." We used to have an old GMC van. It ran well for many years. Everything worked. I looked after it. I had purchased it new, and it was like a friend of the family. I loved it. It had lots of room for bicycles or luggage. If I or someone else made a scratch or a dent in it, I didn't really care. I didn't have to impress anyone. I like myself the way I am and everyone else is entitled to their opinion. So I kept my old vehicle

18

until it fell apart, and I kept the bill collector out of my life. Everything outdates so quickly now that the only thing I am willing to keep buying is information. Futurist Frank Ogden, in *The Last Book You'll Ever Read,* writes: "Your biggest mistake may be your unwillingness to pay for information." Ogden writes that knowledge is doubling every eighteen months, but the pace is increasing faster all the time.

- Make a daily "to do" list to tackle items in order of priority.
- Avoid spending $100 worth of your valuable energy for a 10-cent problem. Enjoy every moment. Stress depletes energy and often results in the inefficient use of time. Ben Franklin said: "Dost thou love life? Then do not squander time, for that is the stuff life is made of."
- Attack a major task or assignment by breaking it down into smaller tasks. This book was written at the pace of just a few pages a day. Set goals that are realistic.
- Balance work with play.
- Be thankful for your comfortable bed, food, water, friends, freedom, a chance to work, and many other blessings!

Controlling Life with Our Mind

Some researchers believe that every thought affects every cell of the body, awake or asleep, 24 hours a day. All of this occurs on a subconscious level, but as the years pass, scientists now find that we can control more and more in our life with our own mind. However, the mind is not only in the head. The mind is throughout the body. Body affects body, brain affects body, and body affects brain.

With excessive uncontrolled worry, people are likely to experience an increase in digestive acids, a tight throat and chest, an increase in heart rate, restless sleep, and perhaps headaches. They may increase their use of drugs, alcohol, food, or cigarettes. In distress, they seek distractions while hoping to numb the pain or provide some pleasure, however temporary.

Yet our natural inborn perfected technology can do much of the searching for the cause of the problem and the perfect solution. These are the unlimited gifts within.

Many years ago, I read research that discovered there is a difference between tears of joy and tears of sadness. Although tears of depression may look the same as tears of laughter, being clear and wet, there is a major unseen difference between the two. Their chemical content is different and varies according to our thoughts. The relatively new field which studies mind and body relationships is called *psychoneuroimmunology.*

One of the pioneers, O. Carl Simonton, M.D., in his popular book, *Getting Well Again,* discusses a variety of positive mental techniques to defend against feelings of hopelessness and even cancer. I gave this book and accompanying audiocassettes to my Aunt Minnie and others. The recommendations of Dr. Simonton have had a remarkable effect in prolonging and adding quality to their lives. It seems so many people who have cancer are those who are always doing wonderful things for other people, but who forget about themselves. I always say: "Love yourself first. Then when your basic needs are satisfied, you can really love and help others."

Simonton discusses such valuable techniques as learning a positive attitude, exercising, regulating your diet, joining an emotional support group of patients who share the same problem, meditating, setting goals, using positive imaging to alter the health of the body or specific parts of the body, visualizing good health and success before it happens, using hypnosis for pain control, using biofeedback, employing therapy to increase feelings of self-worth, and training to cope with stress and anger.

Exercise: Creating Feelings

Remember a time when you felt angry. Create all the details of the event, using all your senses. Notice how you feel. Now remember a time when you felt happy, again using all your senses. Just as we can upset ourselves by reviewing the past over and over, we can choose to feel confident, calm, and happy by selecting memories that inspire those feelings. Moods and attitudes can affect our organs, tissues, our entire physical health. Our immune system is affected by our anger, sadness, and happy states. On the other hand, if you do not feel confident or happy, you can pretend that you are and you can change your emotions. Then you are the master of your own mind.

Prayer and Mind Power

Where the patient has a strong religious faith, prayer may be most beneficial. Some cancer professionals employ psychological techniques in conjunction with standard medical procedures.

The use of "mind power" methods may enhance the benefits of other procedures such as surgery, medication, exercise, and diet. Other benefits may include enhanced rest and better sleep, inner peace, and removal of or a dramatically improved ability to cope with pain. In addition, a more positive outcome from surgery is more likely by instilling confidence in a patient regarding his beliefs about the skills and techniques of the physician coupled with the removal of preoperative fears, stress, and tension.

Direct or indirect suggestions in and out of hypnosis can be most beneficial when used to convince the patient she is capable of rapid recovery and healing. Among many suggestions, medical hypno-therapist, Dr. William J. Bryan, Jr. advocated telling his patients: "You will come out of surgery with a good appetite." The rationale of the suggestion and internal imagery is that if the patient is to come out of surgery with a good appetite, he will have to be alive. Dr. Bryan believed that an operation should not begin unless the patient is convinced of a positive outcome following the operation. Imagine a hypnotherapist in every hospital programming success imagery into every patient who is about to undergo surgery.

Perhaps hospitals could have full-time hypno-technicians to hypnotize patients. Each patient could be given the exact hypnotic suggestions recommended by his or her doctor. Imagine a room filled with people who will undergo the same type of treatment program all feeling optimistic about their future. Do you think that perhaps their body will cooperate better in the healing process?

The Firewalk Experience

Would you walk barefoot over a bed of hot coals or hot stones to build up your confidence? This confidence builder, which is all the rage at some seminars and workshops, borders on a P. T. Barnum publicity stunt. However, if a participant really believes in his mind that he has accomplished the miraculous, then that is wonderful. The experience can boost your confidence—sometimes to a ridiculous extent. Some firewalkers go so far as to believe that they have made themselves immune to fire. Others tell their followers that special powers of immunity to fire have been extended to everyone attending the firewalk event. Regardless of the true worth of this experience, when you believe in yourself, you can do so much more than

21

you ever believed possible. This is not a new development. People have been doing the firewalk for thousands of years.

In 1961, I read about the firewalk experience in D. H. Rawcliffe's excellent reference work, Illusions and Delusions of the Supernatural and the Occult: "...the firewalker induces an autohypnotic state with accompanying analgesia and a psychosomatic modification of the tissues to injury by burning." Rawcliffe adds that part of the preparation for the firewalk may "include fasting, sexual abstinence, prayers, monotonous chanting, exhortations, frenzied rhythmic dancing...The combined effect of many of these initial purification rites must often produce in the walker a highly suggestible trance-like state. There is, however, little indication that the primary function of such preliminaries is anything more than to bring about the expulsion of the walkers' natural fears...a vital point in all types of firewalk. It is necessary to keep one's wits; for poise, correct pacing, and timing are all important...liquors are never taken beforehand...The initial rites therefore play a big role in bolstering up confidence...The feet are actually in contact with the embers less than half a second during each step; this is the secret of the firewalk; and provided the feet are completely dry and free from perspiration, so that no burning ashes adhere to them during the time each foot is in the air, the risks of burning are relatively small...Steadiness in walking is an advantage in order to avoid remaining with the weight on one foot for too long..."

Decades ago and continuing today, some hypnotist entertainers have passed fire under the palm of hypnotized volunteers. As with the firewalk embers, the flame produces a stunning visual effect in a dark room. The volunteer is told to extend his arm straight out, with the palm facing down. The hypnotist strikes up a lighter and passes the flame under the hand with no burning, supposedly due to hypnosis. Genuine as hypnosis is, this stunt is merely an adaptation of a simple magician's trick. If you place your hand through a candle flame, without visiting it too long, you may achieve black fingers, but there will be no burn. Similarly, our entertainer makes sure that the flame from the lighter does not linger long on the volunteer's palm.

Using Hypnosis to Recall the Happy Times

Why not use positive imagery or hypnosis to help people to be thankful for every moment of the gift of life? Hypnosis may be used to help in the recall of all the pleasant memories, the things we have learned, and the thrills we have experienced. Such memories may induce natural chemicals to be released in the body creating a joyous, positive feeling state.

Negative past experiences and memories may be altered to become more positive. Emotional gaps and longings in one's personal history may be patched, altered, redesigned, and changed. Before dying, mental preparation may even begin for the journey to the next world. Different "scripts" of positive suggestions may be composed, depending upon the personal beliefs and the individual desires of each patient. As the most respected medical hypnotherapist Dr. Milton H. Erickson said: "You can practice anything, and master it!" Another wonderful quotation from Dr. Erickson is: "After the rain always comes the sunshine."

The techniques I am about to describe will transform your life. Much of what I discuss also can be done without another person acting as your guide. You will replace the old negative programming with positive affirmations and images. The "mental static" and invisible barriers of the mind can be removed permanently. I am moving slowly because I want you to climb inside my head and understand how I think and how I feel. When you have an understanding and a "feel" for what I write about, you will be able to effortlessly use these invisible gifts which we all possess. You will be able to use the technique at will with precision and joy.

In this book I will use my journeys into the personal memories of my mind to show you how to easily use these processes in your own daily life. Like the pieces of a puzzle, I believe everything will fit together perfectly by the end of this book. I believe that your application of the creative resources and strengths of your inner mind will then be easily and automatically applied to enrich your life.

Countless people have asked me over the past three decades how I became interested in the study of the inner mind, the power of positive thinking, and hypnotic motivation. More importantly, thousands of people have asked me how they can use these wonderful gifts in their own life.

I am a great advocate of positive thinking. However, as Dr.

Albert Ellis and Dr. Robert Harper point out in *A Guide To Successful Marriage,* there are limits to the value of positive thinking: "At the most it may serve as a temporary diversion from your difficulties. It cannot really correct them as long as together with this 'accentuating the positive', you are still unconsciously or unawarely emphasizing the negative."

This quote emphasizes the greater importance of changes within the inner mind. My vision is to share these gifts with as many people as possible. We all have them, but only a small percentage of the population will ever use them. I want you to know and believe that you have these powers inside you and that you easily can use them at will. Once you learn them, my hope is that you will share these techniques with your family, friends, coworkers, and anyone else who will listen.

I say, with confidence, that you can use these techniques on a daily basis to enjoy a healthier, wealthier, and happier life. Perhaps the most wonderful benefit of using these techniques is that when you're satisfied and happy, it is easy for you to love others and help others to enjoy every moment of their lives.

The best way to share these miraculous gifts with you is to start at the beginning. I was born July 1, 1949 in Winnipeg, Manitoba, Canada. For the first 37 years of my life I lived in Winnipeg. I now live in a small seaside community in White Rock, British Columbia, Canada, about 45 minutes from Vancouver. I was the eldest of two boys raised by an Italian father and a Polish mother. Although my parents were born in Canada, my grandparents emigrated from Europe with no money but a strong work ethic.

Having parents from such distinct and opposing nationalities, I experienced, from an early age, a wide variety of society and social characteristics. My Italian background gave me a sense of spontaneity, impulsiveness, and a general joy for life. My Italian relatives taught me warm affection, appreciation of the present, and the exuberance that Italians are well known for. A visit to the Italian side of the family was a loud, boisterous event with grandparents, aunts, and uncles kissing, hugging, and shouting how glad they were to see me. They lived by a simple motto: "Enjoy these precious moments we have together." Every greeting was followed with huge quantities of food and the unending Italian admonishment to eat, eat, and eat some more.

Like many cultures, food was another way to show love. To eat the food was to show appreciation of that love. No wonder I was overweight as a teenager! I hated feeling uncomfortable and habitually buying one size larger. A change of attitude was required. I needed to eat to live, rather than to live to eat.

From my Polish side, I learned how to plan and look forward to the future. Although most of my Polish relatives were not as open in their show of affections as my Italian relatives, they were nonetheless steadfast in their caring and kindness toward me. My Polish grandmother, "Baba," as we have always called her, still lives in Winnipeg. When I think of her, I see two large arms coming to give me a warm and secure hug.

Baba has been known for years as the "world's greatest perogy maker." I remember many family get-togethers, in which Baba would make enough food to feed an army. Chicken, beef, cabbage rolls filled with rice, salads, potatoes and gravy, bread, borscht soup, ice-cream, five or six deserts, soft drinks, milk and, of course, plenty of butter and onions for the perogies. I'm getting hungry just thinking about it. Are you?

Even during short visits to Baba's, I was greeted by those big enveloping arms and a table loaded with food. She would most often say, "You are too small. Eat, I like a big man. You are too skinny."

I appreciated Baba's love for me as expressed through food, but I often had to use self-suggestion and mentally think: "I reject that suggestion; that's ridiculous. My body weight is just right."

Two ideas are important here: First, you reject the negative suggestion. Place a concrete and steel mental wall on top of it. Or place a large black X upon it. Or let it float away in a balloon. Or use some other technique that is effective for you.

Another method is to visualize a large garbage can or incinerator. Imagine that you are placing any negative thoughts that you have about yourself into the garbage can and watch city refuse collectors take them away. The first technique that pops into your head from your inner mind is usually the best one. I'll tell you more about that later.

Secondly, you affirm with a positive suggestion stating what you do want to believe. Remember, with positive suggestions, you always say what you do want, never what you don't want.

The attitude about food that I grew up with was: "Let's celebrate and eat." This attitude is great for the food merchandisers, but it no doubt has led to billions of pounds of extra weight throughout the world. Some people, while trying to control their weight problem while visiting others, have tried another tactic to lose weight. This involves telling your host the following: "I love to visit you, but I find that I eat too much when I come. Your delicious food is so tempting. My doctor says I have to control my weight because it will be easier on my back, to control my blood pressure, etc. I know you love me, but you can show it best by not tempting me with all these wonderful foods."

A more forceful tactic used by some is to say: "Please try your best to help me. If you cannot, I am sorry to say that I will have to reduce the number of visits to your home."

Controlling Weight with Self-Suggestions

When I was a touring hypnotist entertainer in the 1970s, I controlled my weight with a number of self-suggestions. I carried a small one-element burner. In my hotel room, I heated water in a pot, added a little spice, and then ate it from a soup bowl with a spoon. I placed bread upon a plate and ate it with a knife and a fork. For lunch, this would make me feel full and satisfied.

You see, I hypnotized myself to believe that the soup was my favorite soup from the Shanghai Restaurant in Winnipeg, or perhaps a clam chowder. The bread became a wonderful barbecued steak. Believe me, this was an emotionally satisfying meal!

I remember my stage assistant speaking to me while I was eating: "How can you eat that for a meal?" Today, like many people, I eat little meat, so the thought of eating steak is not so appetizing. The types of suggestions that are successful with each individual often change over time.

Addicts are weaned off drugs by a similar process. Addicts may be told under hypnosis that they are feeling the same effects as they would if they took the drug. Therefore, the withdrawal and the drug are eliminated.

A technique that I found useful in my teen years was to look directly into my own eyes while staring into the mirror. With a fixed gaze, you literally can hypnotize yourself and then use this valuable focused attention to plant a positive suggestion into your mind. Using this technique daily over a period of weeks may show startling results.

My Polish grandfather, simply by being in a room, was a hypnotic presence. A philosophical man, he never stopped learning. He could speak several languages. He was an award-winning mink rancher, while it was still fashionable to wear mink in the cold North American winters. Regularly, bits of his advice surface from my unconscious and into my conscious thoughts. This reminds me of the Woody Allen movie, Oedipus Wrecks in *New York Stories*, in which his deceased mother appears like King Kong in the distance always giving him advice.

Negative parental voices can be devastating to people. We can spend a lifetime walking around with needless guilt, worries, and fears, which were planted deep in the unconscious mind at an early age. Memories of *positive* parental images and voices can be remarkably uplifting during times of setbacks and obstacles.

Most parents, with the limited knowledge that they all have and with the excess baggage they are still carrying from their childhood, do the best they can. Through the use of these wonderful inborn and natural techniques I am about to describe, I believe that I have overcome most of the limitations of my childhood.

I feel happy, healthy, and successful almost 100 percent of the time. I never feel that life owes me any more than I have. Sometimes I prefer alternate outcomes, but they really are not all that important to me. I never feel bored. I can entertain myself for hours reading, gardening, writing, visiting beautiful places, meeting interesting people, seeking out opportunities for growth and discovery, and enjoying nature.

Affirmations from a Polish Grandfather

Here are some of the positive affirmations that I allow to remain and echo in my mind. They come from my Polish grandfather:

"My best friend is a book."

"You have to have a goal. Life is like a ship. If you do not have a destination in mind, the wind will blow you this way and that way. You have to have a goal."

"You have to make a decision, but the decision has to be the right one. The decision has to be a calculated one. If you make too many wrong decisions, you are finished."

"Most important is the respect for the dignity of the individual."

My Polish grandfather took courses into his eighties. He gave my brother Dave and me a set of encyclopedias for Christmas in 1961. He taught me the importance of education and organization. But, most importantly, by his own actions, he showed me the pleasure of hard work and the value of education. He showed me how to develop concentration and focus, which is so important for success.

I have had to develop a balance between the "have fun today" attitude of my Italian side and the "let's work and plan for tomorrow" attitude of my Polish side. In the past, my dichotomous ancestry has led to guilty thoughts: "I should be working instead of playing" or "I should be playing instead of working." Today, however, I believe I have nearly solved the problem. I normally do not do work unless it is like play, unless I enjoy it. My work is in large part my play, because I enjoy it so thoroughly. Each day, I live more and more in the moment, enjoying life more and more every day.

I had to learn to avoid feeling guilty about having fun during free time. I had to learn not to turn everything into a goal achievement task. So now, most of the time, I do only what I enjoy doing. This attitude keeps my energy high.

Liking What You Do—And Making Money at It

Many people say that they go to work to earn a living and that they do not like their work. One article I read claimed that 80 percent of Canadians dislike their work. If someone came to me and told me that he did not like his work, I would hypnotize him to go inside his unconscious mind to find out what he really would like to do. Once he finds a particular hobby or interest, a part-time occupation may start and develop into enjoyable, honest, income-producing self-employment.

To me, good health, happiness, and helping others to achieve good health and happiness is everything that I strive to achieve. Many people I have encountered in my life have told me that they needed more money to be happy. Liberace once said that he has been poor and he has been rich and that being rich was more fun.

When I was a teenager, I went through a few years thinking:

"Money is not important. All they want is money. Money was a 'dirty' word."

A huge percentage of divorces occur because of money problems. Medical treatment or education may be denied because of a lack of money. Some people starve because of a lack of money. I quickly learned that money is important, that it can give me freedom to achieve my goals and to help others to achieve their goals.

Many therapists and wonderful healers have had to change careers because they didn't make enough money from their services. To be a success in my line of work or any other form of work that you love to do requires entrepreneurial skills: such as identifying a worthwhile product or service and learning business basics, marketing skills, and negotiation skills.

The best source of entrepreneurial training assistance that I can recommend is E. Joseph Cossman's books and seminars. Joe has helped thousands of people change their careers, and many have become millionaires while doing what they love to do. One of his books, co-authored with William A. M. Cohen, is called *Making It*.

Joe possesses the charisma and the magic of a master communicator and teacher. He has a remarkable ability to help you to believe in yourself and in your abilities. He has a rare gift for clear, concise communication, often educating with personal stories and metaphors. It has been said that top executives have what is call Executive ESP. In Joe's case, he always seems to know what you're thinking. He would have been a great mind reader, hypnotist, or therapist. He also has an extraordinary ability to counsel others in not only business, but personal aspects of life as well.

In 1994, Joe and his wife Pearl joined me for a vacation on Vancouver Island. I enjoyed watching Joe converse with strangers. Within seconds, he had his listener smiling and eager to help him or to continue the conversation. Joe has a gift for bringing out the best in even strangers, in minutes. To me, Joe is a best friend and mentor. Students of Joe's home study entrepreneurship training program do not require a high level of education. As Joe says: "You can work from a kitchen table starting your business with less than $50."

Joe Cossman started at the bottom and learned a simple step-by-step formula for success. He also has a sincere desire to help others to achieve happiness in their careers. There are thousands of systems available that do not work. However, if you are hungry for success in starting your own business or for financial independence, you can join thousands of others who Joe has helped. You can reach Joe at P.O. Box 4480, Palm Springs, California 92263. Tell him Romane sent you and that you want help to start your own business making money doing what you love to do.

Stop Smoking with Hypnosis

Stop smoking programs are one of the most successful and most gratifying parts of my business. Hypnosis is highly effective for smoking cessation, especially when combined with traditional medical and psychological methods. At the 1993 Annual Convention of the National Guild of Hypnotists, Dr. Masud Ansari stated, "The most effective and short-cut therapy to stop nicotine dependency is through hypnosis."

I love to help people, especially to help them stop smoking. Once in a small town grocery store, I sadly watched a young father buy two cartons of poisonous cigarettes, while the son he was holding was wearing worn out shoes with enormous holes.

In Calgary, a woman told me: "My husband's doctor told me that my husband would be dead today if he had not come to your seminar." Today, most of my clients seem to decide to attend my seminars because they have been referred by others who have been successful at my seminars.

One mentor of mine used to say that if you give people what they need, then you will be successful. I found out the hard way that you have to give people what they want. I originally hoped to give full day or several evening seminars for people wishing to stop smoking. This obviously would be more effective. However, few people would come, because most people are too "busy" to spend time looking after themselves. In fact, most people are too busy in their lives to maintain the close relationships that they desire.

My self-improvement seminars are vital not only to my business but to my well-being. I love helping people. I especially enjoy hypnotizing others to help them to stop smoking, lose weight, or to maximize their potential. Anyone who uses these techniques will likely be healthier and happier and live longer.

When I help parents stop smoking, stay alive, and be healthier, I am also helping thousands of children. Children in smokers' homes have as much as 17 times the respiratory diseases as children in nonsmokers' homes. These children also have more lead in their bloodstream than children who live near a smelter. Finally, when I help smokers kick the habit, I am helping to clean the environment. No wonder my stop smoking seminars are among my favorite.

One way to stop smoking is to place a couple of dozen or so cigarette butts into a sealed bottle for a few days. Then open the bottle and breathe the air. Think about how that foul odor makes your body feel. A good time to do this is before sleep.

If that is not enough motivation to quit smoking, let me relate a true story of a real estate agent who was a smoker. Apparently a client was ready to purchase a property, but when the real estate agent lit up his cigarette, the client was offended. The client promptly left the company of the real estate agent and the agent lost a $7,000 commission. There was even a case of a wife suing her husband because his smoking made their dog sick.

Now here's a true story about a deceased 74-year-old Romanian chain-smoking millionaire. His will left his fortune to his wife with a conditional clause. To inherit his money, she had to smoke five cigarettes a day, "for the woman nagged me about every cigarette I ever smoked, and she is going to pay for it now!" His 80-year-old widow is contesting the will as "unreasonable."

How to Become a Millionaire

Here is my formula for how to become a millionaire:

1. Choose what you love to do that fulfills people's *wants*, not necessarily their *needs*. Hopefully, you will fulfill both a want and a need.

2. Spend your money on knowledge and education, not expensive cars, opulent apartments, over-priced vacations, and other fads. How much you save can be more important than how much you earn.

3. Spend your time with successful people, positive people. Steer clear of negative people or anyone who thinks making profits is a negative thing.

4. Secure employment to work directly with highly successful people, even if you have to first offer your services for free.

5. Read books and listen to lectures, cassettes, and videos of leaders

in their field. Take their seminars, too. If the seminars are out of your price range, offer to work at the seminar for free.

6. Persist. Never give up.

A client of mine once sent the following quotation (author unknown) to me: "I shall pass through this world but once. Any good, therefore, that I can do, or any kindness that I can show to any human being, let me do it now. Let me not defer nor neglect it, for I shall not pass this way again."

Put Your Imagination to Work

During my early childhood years, my family struggled in poverty. My father labored on the railroad, while my mother worked occasionally as a waitress. My father collected bags of pop bottles from the streets and ditches for a little extra money. Up until the age of seven, I was an only child. I was shy and often alone. I invented my own games to entertain myself. Using my imagination was good practice for my later work with alternative methods of health care such as hypnosis and creative imagery. The imagination assists you in making better use of various techniques such as healing imagery, creative visualization, concentration, mental rehearsal, mental discipline, successful mind programming, focusing, and mental training.

We use visualization skills every day. For example, when we daydream about an upcoming vacation or mentally plan a trip from one location to another, we are visualizing. Efficient visualization with an accompanying altered state of consciousness is usually characterized by:

1. Relaxation
2. Focused concentration
3. Emptying the mind

You may choose to use these skills to become a winner, to achieve maximum performance in any area of life. The skills may be used to reach goals. A Hitler or Stalin can use them as can a doctor, a patient, a president, or a saint. Adults or children can use them. However, anyone who does use these healing techniques should be aware that he has control over the images in his mind. In other words, this state of mind is totally safe. You can also leave this mental state anytime you wish, stopping or leaving any mental daydream behind you.

Being alone a lot, I can remember being in touch with that little inner voice we all receive when we are born. The answers lie within us. All we need to do is look, listen, and trust. I am referring to the voice of intuition, inner knowledge, and wisdom. These are standard items in the professional hypnotherapist's toolbox.

4

Hypnosis: Learning to Use Your Natural Gift

In 1955, the British Medical Association reported its approval of hypnosis as a valuable tool in the treatment of psychoneuroses and for hypnoanesthesia in surgery. In 1958, the American Medical Association approved the use of hypnosis as a scientific tool. Today, this incredible gift is used in countries worldwide. Physicians, psychiatrists, psychologists, dentists, nurses, ministers, social workers, teachers, the police, and many other professionals help patients to release these natural inborn healing methods.

Unfortunately, due to an inappropriate use of the word hypnosis by various fiction writers, hypnosis is often confused with black magic, voodoo, witchcraft, and Satanism. It is amazing how many otherwise intelligent individuals can confuse hypnosis with the supernatural and the occult. This negative aura still hovers over hypnosis in spite of millions attesting to the benefits in overcoming pain, in getting rid of negative habits or "mental blocks," in making personality changes, and in enhancing creativity.

The methods I advocate are natural gifts of the Creator. I believe that anyone who does not use these great gifts is missing a major gift of strength, given to everyone at birth. Many problems can be solved with this gift. Hypnosis is a powerful tool that is a living example of: "God helps those who help themselves."

It Began with the Amazing Hypno-Coin

As a young boy, I loved to write away for mail offers. I wrote away for memberships to coin and stamp collection companies and dozens of different mail offers. I would wait eagerly for the postman each day.

My first recollection of anything to do with hypnosis was when I was just nine years old. I read an advertisement in a magazine and immediately sent fifty cents for my "amazing hypno-coin." It was a plastic spiral, about the size of a large old silver dollar. The modus-operandi was to hold the hypno-coin between the thumb and index finger while turning the thumb and finger left and right, back and forth. This gave the illusion that the spiral was drawing you inwards and served as a point of fixation. Focusing attention is critical to hypnosis. Whether the point of fixation is a light, a speck on a ceiling, lying on a couch looking up at a corner on a ceiling where the walls all meet, a coin, a ring, a happy face on a thumb for a child, or just focusing on your breath as it goes in and out, you can bring about a relaxing state of inner peace.

The hypno-coin sparked my first fascination with hypnosis and the mind. I studied brain power because I had an intrinsic interest in the mysteries and marvels of our capabilities. In fact, I studied so much in those days that my Uncle Neno used to call me "The Professor." Just recalling those days now fires me up with the enthusiasm of youth. In short, from the age of nine, my main interest in life was the study of the human mind and its potential.

In 1956, when mail order hypno-coin were popular, the book The Search For Bridey Murphy by Morey Bernstein was a best-seller. This book described memories of a previous life recalled under hypnosis. I experimented with my hypno-coin on my unsuspecting little brother, Dave, who was only two years old at the time. My brother is now a successful businessman and my closest friend. Dave owns Pro-Auto Ltd. and Pro-Body Parts Ltd. with locations in Vancouver, Toronto, Winnipeg, and Calgary. He imports millions of dollars of parts and resells them in Canada and other countries. He also is involved in real estate and other ventures. Could it be that this early experience with hypnosis helped him on the road to a happy and successful life? I can only hope the answer is YES! (By the way, he also completed Joe Cossman's course.)

When we were growing up, I gave my brother a lot of advice such as "the most successful and happiest are not necessarily the most knowledgeable, but those who have a positive mental attitude will develop success and friendships." I don't know anyone who has as many friends as Dave. When good advice is given to children at an early age, the imprint capacity is strongest and positive suggestions create the greatest benefits. However, as with most things in life, there is good and bad about this imprint power. An example of bad inprinting is the mass brainwashing used by Hitler on Germany's youth.

Earl Nightingale, author of the popular Lead The Field audiocassette series, uses the magic word "attitude" throughout his writings. Earl's advice is that the world will respond to us according to our attitude, a simple law of cause and effect.

Futurist Frank Ogden writes in *The Last Book You'll Ever Read*: "Hire on attitude alone. Credentials are from the past, and past skills are obsolete."

In a lecture at the 1993 Annual Convention of the National Guild of Hypnotists, speaker Ross G. Brochhagen noted a 1985 survey by Allen Cox. In the survey of 1,173 CEOs, 85 percent said that their success was based upon their attitude. Only 15 percent said that their success was based upon education and experience. Surprisingly, in the area of budgeting, it was stated that corporations only spend 5 percent of their budget on attitude development and 95 percent on education and experience.

I am always reminding my own children to have a positive attitude. The mirrors in our home each have a small sign with one word written on them: "Attitude." I have found that indirect advice works best. What my children—Vance, 12; Elizabeth, 13; and Diana, 15—see me do is far more powerful in establishing healthy ways of thinking, feeling, and behaving than anything I might say. For example, I may leave a book, such as *The Magic of Believing* by Claude M. Bristol, on a table. I do not necessarily expect my children to read it, but I want them to see the cover. They then know that my mind is focusing on the positive. This indirect suggestion is far more powerful than me saying, "Be positive." There are times when my children, like all children, will argue and shout at each other or feel a lack of confidence. However, I know that as they grow older all the positive advice and indirect suggestions that I have given them will materialize and surface to help them live healthier, happier, and more successful lives.

Sometimes I am more direct as when I gave Diana a copy of Dale Carnegie's classic, *How To Win Friends And Influence People*, which has sold more than 15 million copies. A few months later, Diana was out cycling and noticed an old copy of *The Dale Carnegie Course in Effective Speaking and Human Relations* at a garage sale. I was thrilled when she brought it home as a gift for me.

Hypnotic Susceptibility in Children

When I hypnotized Dave, I was unaware, of course, that such a young child would be difficult to hypnotize. In addition, my techniques were limited at best. Although young children may be hypnotized quite easily because of their tremendous imagination skills, psychological research has determined that the age span of 8 to 12 years is the peak of hypnotic susceptibility in children. Hypnotherapists agree that childhood is a constant state of hypnosis.

There are numerous textbooks and workshops that focus on the uses of hypnosis with children. Today, there are specialists who work exclusively in the area of hypnosis with children. Two related texts are *Clinical Hypnosis with Children*, edited by William C. Wester, Ed.D. and Donald J. O'Grady, Ph.D., and *Hypnosis and Hypnotherapy with Children,* by G. Gail Gardner, Ph.D. and Karen Olness, M.D. Hypnosis often is used with children to address psychological and behavior problems, to eliminate habits, to improve recovery from surgery, to control pain, and to enhance learning.

As a youngster, my cautious and future-oriented Polish side told me to study and learn as much about hypnosis and mind power techniques as I could. And I did. I was so fascinated with brain power that from the age of nine, I spent the following three years reading and studying everything I could get my hands on about the subject. Looking back, it seems humorous that at such a young age I would be studying and researching hypnosis so diligently. Although, I must say that I am glad that I had a major interest. I always feel sorry for someone who says: "I have no interests. I'm bored."

I see the same diligence in my son Vance, who at the age of nine was studying books on animation art. He attended comic conventions, clipboard in hand, price values memorized. He perused comics, talked to artists, visited art studios, and a reporter had asked him for an interview to write a newspaper feature! Since he was a young child, he has spent all his spare time drawing. He *loves* drawing, and he says he wants a career in animation. Today, at age 12, his main interests are computers and the Internet.

Vance rarely uses any medication. He often has heard me say: "I would rather do it the natural way, with my mind," and he often does. Sometimes he even reminds me of a technique at the appropriate time of need.

Children can easily be instructed in techniques of relaxation, concentration, and imagination. Children, as well as adults, may use these techniques to feel a sense of self-mastery, confidence, and control. Performance may be enhanced in school, at sports, and practically any other area. Whatever you do, you can do it better with practical mind-training techniques.

After attaining a relaxed state of mind, with the methods in this book, children may be asked to use all their senses to vividly *imagine themselves performing successfully* in school (confidence, powerful concentration skills, effortless recall abilities during exams) as well as in music, art, or sports. Positive affirmations can be repeated over and over for added effect. Quiet meditative music also may be played to create the focused mood of relaxation and concentration.

In June 1994, my family and I held a stop smoking seminar in Vancouver, British Columbia. My son showed all the adults in the audience how to tense up their muscles and release the tension for total relaxation. I'm sure the audience will always remember Vance. Here was a nine year old in a black tuxedo, red bow-tie, and red cumberbund showing them how to have a more relaxed life without a need to smoke. The indirect suggestion that I wanted to convey was: "If a young boy can do that, you can too."

My two daughters, Diana and Elizabeth, also help with my seminars or office work. They are exposed to my way of thinking, and I hope they are able to absorb some ideas without conscious effort on their part. Many of the techniques are simply an attitude or way of thinking about life. Often my employees have said that their self-image and their attitude about work and life completely changed by working with me. Similarly, I greatly appreciate learning from everyone with whom I connect, whether family, employee, client, or stranger. I believe there is something to learn from everyone.

If a challenge arises in my own life, I try to disregard the problem and focus upon the solution. I won't say my way of thinking is best for everyone, but it sure works for me and thousands of people who have taken my programs. There are many roads to happiness. However, many people come to me with no map whatsoever in mind. I give them a route to follow. If one method does not work for that individual, there is *always* another route to follow. If I am stuck, I just ask my unconscious mind to give me an answer. In seconds, I can self-induce a relaxation of my mind and body. Then, I present the need to my unconscious mind and request a solution. *The most important principle is to trust the unconscious to deliver the answer.*

As of 1996, none of my children receive an allowance. We pay for all of their necessities, and they live comfortably. However, just like the real world, they must earn all their own spending money. I usually have a job for them if they want to help or if they need money. Diana really likes to work at my seminars. However, seeing the self-employed entrepreneur in me, she started her own business a few years ago. She decided that she wanted to represent Caeran's environmentally friendly cleaning products as well as Regal Greeting Cards & Gifts. As a result, she designed her own business card and had it printed with both the Regal and Caeran logos. Both local papers published feature articles on her entrepreneurship.

Hypnotherapy: Using Inner Strengths to Heal

Today there is increasing interest in alternative methods of health care and healing. Hypnotherapy is one of these and represents an easy and safe method to achieve maximum use of inner strengths and resources.

My family and I are also great believers in muscle massage. We have our own massage table, and we often give each other a massage to eliminate muscle tension. For several decades, I have worked with hypnosis, mental imagery, behavior modification, and progressive relaxation techniques. I have discovered that you can eliminate or at least diminish many problems by showing someone how to control physical tension and mental stress. By adding a dash of self-esteem building and self-love, forgiveness of self and others, most clients will be far healthier mentally as well as physically.

I have found that there is some tension that responds much better to massage, shiatzu, or chiropractic care than to hypnosis. Our entire family visits a chiropractor for regular care and spinal alignment.

Give Yourself a Regular Mind Tune-up

Hypnotherapy is an excellent tool to help you reshape personality, eliminate unhealthy habits, or establish new healthy habits. Mind training methods can help you be your best at anything you do. For more serious problems, you may also participate in hypnoanalysis, which helps you discover the root cause of problems. Some massage practitioners combine massage with hypnosis to create hypno-massage. They add relaxing music and aromatherapy to create a pleasant experience that is even more therapeutic.

Many massage therapists visit offices during the day to give brief neck, back, and shoulder massages. Perhaps some day a short break with meditation or hypnosis will be commonplace as well. A "relaxation break" is far healthier than a smoke or coffee break.

You Have the Gift, Too

It's true that the Creator-given, inborn skills you are about to master cannot do everything, but they can help you to do almost anything better. We all have these gifts and talents, and I would love to share my years of study with you to show you how you can use them, too.

Ever since childhood, I have wanted a career that would allow me "to help others." Many people have said to me: "You have a gift to help others." When I give a private session, a show, or a seminar, I give my last bit of energy. Sometimes, I ask a member of the audience afterwards if they recognized that I was drained and they never do. I always try to appear full of energy until the end, otherwise I worry that I might undo some of the good that I have created in their mind. I do my best to give 110 percent at all times.

However, anyone can help others as I do. By devoting enough study time, combined with the practical experience necessary to sharpen skills, what I do can be learned by almost anyone. I say this because over the years many people have assumed that I possess some type of inborn ability. No, my skills are all learned.

On this subject, I recommend a great book called *If You Meet The Buddha On The Road, Kill Him*, by Sheldon B. Kopp. I never want to see anyone dependent upon me, although I'm happy to be a temporary crutch for someone. My seminars, my writings, and my recordings are great, but each person must use these tools in a way that best fits his or her individual nature. Again, your unconscious mind will be your ultimate guide.

Too much dependence already is fostered by some therapists. The most evil form of dependence control are cults. There are more than 5,000 known cults in America. Their ability to mold the mind of their devotees is so great that even with knowledge of mind control methods, association with them can be dangerous. I have heard of mind control experts joining cults to investigate them and then being convinced to become permanent members. I expand on this topic in another chapter.

How to Make Hypnosis Work for You

Although hundreds of thousands of people have come to my presentations, it is most interesting to note that different people have dramatically different reactions to my work. For example, a few weeks after one seminar, someone telephoned me to say that she and several of her friends had all stopped smoking at the seminar. They raved for several minutes about how successful the seminar was. Later, that very same day, a lady telephoned me to say that the seminar did absolutely nothing for her and her friend, and that she felt that the program was a total waste of time. I interpret this to mean that the last two folks just were not ready to stop smoking at this time in their lives. Perhaps too much stress was occurring in their lives at the time or perhaps they just had so many problems that they needed private one-on-one counseling.

However, just having to rush to the seminar can upset someone enough that they may find it more difficult to concentrate. The reasons are unlimited. *When hypnosis does not work, this is most likely due to the fact that the session occurred at the wrong time, the wrong method was used, the wrong hypnotist was employed, or the suggestions were not repeated often enough.*

All hypnotists are far from being the same in demeanor, voice tone, knowledge, cleanliness, friendliness, and in ability to inspire confidence and trust. Age or sex of the hypnotist may even have an effect on the success of the therapy. There are a huge number of variables that will affect the success rate. Once a client complained of his difficulty stopping smoking after attending one of my seminars. Wanting to help him, I said: "Can you suggest anything that might improve my program?" He said: "Make it work." Often

41

people will think of hypnosis as a magical method to "fix" them like a toaster or a TV. In addition, they want a lifetime guarantee of success no matter what happens in their life.

On the positive side, when someone "hangs in there" and is persistent, they are highly likely to be successful. If results are not positive, sometimes there is just a clash of the personalities of the hypnotist and the client. Changing the location; the gender, attitude, or voice of the therapist; the room temperature; the comfort of the chair can make success happen.

Often *permanent* success does occur *in only one session*. However, even in the cases of instant success, I recommend repeating the session many times for added reinforcement and lasting results.

People often will travel thousands of miles to see an "expert." Sometimes the expert is right around the corner, but he may not be perceived as the expert because he is so close in terms of miles. Dr. William J. Bryan, Jr. used to say, "The expert is always 50 miles away. A prophet can be just a carpenter in his own town."

The *Bible* puts it another way: "A prophet is not without honor, save in his own country, and in his own house." (Matthew, 8:57)

Fearing the Power of the Brain

By the time I was 12, I was regularly hypnotizing my friends. This went on throughout my teens. The reaction I received was most often encouraging. Many of my friends were not only interested, they were *fascinated.* They found it comical, fun, and inspiring. However, some were skeptical about it and some even feared it.

Many times people have been afraid to look in my eyes because they fear I will use my hypnotic skills to overpower them. I'll never forget performing as a young hypnotist at the Lyric Theatre in Beausejour, Manitoba. As I walked up the center aisle to begin my presentation, a man seated in the first seat on the aisle turned his head away and placed his hand over his eyes. At first I thought such people were teasing me, then I realized they actually were afraid of hypnosis and me.

Fear and imagination combined are powerful forces. I am reminded of a story I used to tell my audiences when I was in my teens and early twenties. I would say: "Imagine that we have a 12-foot plank, which is 1-foot wide and thick enough to never bend or break.

Imagine maintaining your balance and walking from one end of the plank to the other. That's easy."

"Now imagine that we take that same plank and place it between two tall buildings. It is a pleasant warm day and there is no wind. Unless you were a steeplejack, would you feel just as comfortable walking across the plank? Actually, if you can walk across it on the floor, it is no different to walk across it while it is suspended between the two tall buildings. However, there is a difference. Our active imagination and fear mechanism begin to work together. We think and visualize losing our balance, falling, and being killed. If we walked across that plank, chances are good that our imagination would make us so nervous that we would make our thoughts come true and actually lose our balance and fall."

As is clearly stated in the *Bible,* that which we fear comes upon us. We tend to attract the things which we fear. Similarly, if we expect good fortune, good health, love, financial success, and all things positive, we will radiate more confidence and love and good things are more likely to happen in our life.

When we do not understand something, our imagination always can make it bigger and scarier. Besides using the great gift of imagination for art, music, dance, scientific discovery, and invention, we may use our imagination to change our thoughts, feelings, and behavior. All we have to do is focus the mind, relax the body, and repeatedly impress carefully planned positive suggestions into the inner mind. The more imaginative senses we use (seeing, hearing, feeling, tasting, touching), the more powerful the changes. The motivation or strength of the desire to change is critical. If we generate highly emotional suggestions that evoke strong feelings, the changes will be faster and stronger. Repetition of positive imagery is also important for permanence.

If you imagine that you are attractive or competent, you will bring out the best in yourself. When you give someone a compliment, you may change their mental state and feelings because of the combination of the power of your words and their imagination. You become a hypnotist with your choice of words, positive or negative. Similarly, what you say mentally to yourself and what you think about yourself creates your future, how you act, who you meet, who you marry, the type of work you choose.

43

I graduated in 1967 from Vincent Massey Collegiate in Winnipeg. The caption next to my picture in the yearbook said, "most likely to be a hypnotherapist." While my friends played hockey or football, I studied and practiced hypnotherapy. In my studies of brain power, I learned how to improve my concentration and relaxation skills. I also was easily able to overcome my incessant nail-biting habit.

While in high school, I read the book, *A Practical Guide To Better Concentration,* by Melvin Powers and Robert S. Starrett. The cover of the book shows a sketch of a man in a suit jacket with his head tilted down as if reading a book. The man's right hand is in a loosely closed fist with the index finger resting on the chin and the thumb is along the right jawbone. He epitomizes concentration.

After reading this book, I would lie down in bed at night and mentally relax my body from the bottom of my feet to the top of my head. I would then imagine myself in the same position as the man on the book cover. The two separate mental pictures I projected into my mind were (1) myself with perfect concentration while seated in the classroom and (2) myself with perfect concentration while seated at home at my desk. In my mental imagery, I saw myself with perfect concentration in the same pose as the man on the book cover. The results were phenomenal! Whenever I sat down to study, all I had to do was place my right hand upon my chin and my concentration was powerful in the classroom or at home.

Again, these outstanding results may require repeated success imagery over weeks, but the magical results are well worth the time. You are programming your inner mind to automatically respond with success when it comes up against a real world situation where you need to perform at your best. The axiom is the subconscious does not know the difference between an imaginary success experience and a real one.

Simple techniques are often the best. The mind will respond to positive or negative suggestions, so it is important whenever and wherever possible to only feed your mind what you do want to happen in your life, never what you don't want to happen. I am a great believer in avoiding negative suggestions such as "I will not do such and such." Always suggest in words and pictures what you do want, not what you don't want.

5

Breaking Bad Habits

In the 1960s, when I listed myself in the Yellow Pages of the Winnipeg telephone directory, I was the only listing under hypnotist. Now there are thousands of trained hypnotherapists in the United States and Canada alone who use hypnosis with patients on a daily basis. Hypnosis is popular worldwide because it works so well to overcome so many human difficulties.

Occasionally I will give a limited number of negative fear-inducing suggestions, but only as a last resort. One client of mine had a habit of drinking several large bottles of cola soft drink every day. When she imagined that snakes were inside the bottle, she promptly overcame the habit. During hypnosis, questions directed to her subconscious mind told us that negative suggestions would work with her addiction.

In my mid-teens, I had a habit of biting my fingernails. Motivated by upcoming TV appearances, which would zoom in and focus on my hands, I gave myself a suggestion while in self-hypnosis, that was 100 percent visual. I pictured my nails as already long, focusing exclusively on the end result. I stopped biting my nails immediately, following only one night of a few minutes of hypnotic self-suggestion. This happened to work faster than improving my concentration, which took about two weeks for truly noticeable improvement. After four weeks, my concentration had improved dramatically.

There are many sources for information about brain power. I recommend the books of Melvin Powers, who has done a lot of good work in the field of hypnosis. He has a large collection of publications, which are distributed by the millions to book stores and via mail order. To order his catalog, write: Melvin Powers, 12015 Sherman Road., North Hollywood CA 91605, phone: (818) 765-8529. Another good source is the work of Dr. William J. Bryan, Jr., M.D., who was founder of the American Institute of Hypnosis in Los Angeles. He originated the idea that treatment rooms can be electronically wired so that several patients can be seen at the same time by one physician. With a central control room and patients with headphones in several different rooms, recorded messages can be played back to clients simultaneously. Although patients are initially seen privately, in later sessions patients receive reinforcement suggestions in hypnosis via cassette tape. In one room a patient can be improving his memory to do better on an exam, another might be overcoming a temper problem, yet in another room a patient can be going through a past life regression.

The doctors at the institute watch the patients on separate monitors, while varying the suggestions according to their reactions. There are many hypnotists today who use these central control rooms for treating several patients simultaneously. The hypnotist will likely have hundreds of different recordings to be matched up with the individual needs of each client. These recordings are not meant to replace the hypnotist. As Dr. Bryan said: "You have to know what you are doing. What if the tape machine breaks down?"

I still have a set of more than 200 original Dr. Bryan cassettes known as the *Dr. Bryan Master Tapes*. Each tape was designed for application to many different problem areas. In the 1970s, the *Bryan Master Tapes* were sold as a set for $10,000 U.S. During his life, Dr. Bryan trained thousands of doctors to use hypnosis, edited a hypnosis journal, and regularly organized tours to different countries for the purpose of visiting foreign hypnosis centers.

Dr. Bryan was well known for his simple demonstrations of negative suggestions. For example, he would tell an audience to try not think of a pink elephant. Of course, the harder you try not to think of something, the more you will think about it. Dr. Bryan would say that the best way to get rid of the elephant is to think of something else, a giraffe for example. Similarly, a theatrical hypnotist will say: "Try *hard*, to pull your clasped hands apart, but they lock tighter and tighter." Sometimes, Dr. Bryan would advise a lawyer to omit saying that his client is not guilty, but instead to speak of the client as being innocent. Again, focus on what you do want, not what you don't want. Forget the problem; focus on the solution and what you can do.

Instant Change

Many clients come to a therapist, particularly hypnotists, with a desire for instant change. Once a tense client came into my office walking at a rapid pace. He handed me a small sheet of paper with a written note from his psychiatrist; it was a referral for relaxation therapy. The client then rapidly plopped down into my big, soft black leather armchair and shouted in an urgent voice: "Hurry up and relax me!" I was caught a little off guard and knew immediately my work would take longer than the client expected. Those who are in a hurry usually take longer.

Much of my work has been through referrals. Sometimes I ask a group at my stop smoking seminars: "How many of you came here tonight because you know someone who has been helped at my seminars?" As many as 90 percent raise their hands. Testimonials of friends has far more credibility than advertising in my profession.

I also agree with the famous car dealer Cal Worthington who said on a television talk show several years ago: "If they don't like you, they are not going to buy from you." Sales superstar Joe Girard says the average person can refer you to 250 people, because that is the average number of people who come to a funeral. Every year I hold seminars in 50 to 60 cities. The cooler months are my busiest times; in January, I may appear in 25 cities.

Haste Makes Waste Even in Hypnosis

My first job was at the age of five. I lived next to the Solo grocery store in Winnipeg, and I asked the owner, Andy, for a job. He offered me a job to cut his grass with hand clippers along the side of the store facing the alley. When I think of it, this job never really needed to be done, but he offered to help me out. I was thrilled to be earning 25 cents per hour. At 5 cents each, that was a lot of popsicles!

When I was in my early teens, I worked for Andy again as a grocery delivery boy. I had a large basket on my bike, and I delivered the groceries as fast as my legs could pedal. About the second or third time out, I slipped and crashed the bike on the road. Eggs, milk, bread, and everything littered the road. Andy calmly said to me, "Were you in a hurry?"

I said, "Yes."

He simply said, "Haste makes waste." He did not have to say any more. From then on, I took my time and never spilled the groceries again.

It is commonly known that people who lose weight slowly are far more likely to keep the weight off permanently. This allows time for new habits to be established. Some physicians claim that it takes one to two years for new eating habits to be permanently established. However, when clients hear that they have to work at change, they often give up. Many people will choose to spend their time being entertained rather than spend time attending a wellness program. And if I tell people that eliminating a problem may take more than one session, often they will give up even making an attempt to eliminate the problem.

The first person I deeply hypnotized was a schoolmate named Helmut. At the tender age of 13, we attended our first staged hypnotist act. Helmut volunteered to be a part of the act, but was rejected by the hypnotist as not being susceptible to hypnosis. Helmut was, however, in somewhat of a daze, it seemed. When he returned to his seat, he sat on the fedora that belonged to a man seated next to him. The hat was flattened, and Helmut received an angry look from his neighbor.

I was positive that I had the ability to hypnotize Helmut and, after the show, we went back to another friend's house where I quickly accomplished just that. Helmut, I found out, was a good subject who was capable of experiencing a deep somnambulistic state. With his permission, I easily conditioned him to enter deep hypnosis at the snap of a finger or at the sound of the words, "Spanish Armada."

This worked so well that I unintentionally hypnotized Helmut while quietly whispering the words, "Spanish Armada," over 50 feet away. I quickly discovered that the subconscious has far more acute hearing than the conscious mind.

Helmut was known as a bit of a ruffian in those days and was easily provoked into a little horse play. My hypnotism worked even when he was on the verge of coming to blows with others. I would simply snap my fingers and the tough Helmut would fall to the ground like a stack of cards, leaving his would-be opponent surprised and probably grateful.

One year Helmut neglected his school work and came to me a couple of days before his final exams for an emergency hypnosis session. He hoped hypnosis would help him pass his exams. Unfortunately, Helmut failed the exam. If we had begun his hypnotherapy several weeks earlier, he may well have passed that year.

Hypnosis can help students in areas such as concentration, memory, overcoming exam jitters, motivation to study, self-esteem enhancement, and sports. Although these applications have shown improvement with one hypnosis session, more outstanding and more permanent results usually occur only with several sessions. A cassette tape of the session is also helpful for reinforcement at home. Tapes greatly increase the likelihood of permanent success.

I was one of the first hypnotists to make hypnosis recordings. In the 1960s psychologists at the University of Manitoba told me that therapy had to be conducted face to face with a therapist. Supposedly, change was not possible through home study recordings. How times have changed. Today a vast supply of therapeutic recordings are being mass merchandised by psychologists and medical doctors for help with practically any human problem you can imagine—from enhancing motivation and understanding of the mind to learning new attitudes or skills. These recordings are most valuable when used as reinforcement.

As responsibility shifts more and more to the patient with assigned books, tapes, and projects, the patient also learns to realize he is in control of his destiny. He learns to feel empowered to find the solution to his problems without outside help. The patient can learn how to do research to find his own solutions. The answers to eliminate a problem or at least to learn to cope with it are available. On the other hand, blaming (and not taking responsibility) makes you feel like a victim and makes you feel disempowered.

Above all, the patient must learn that no strange force controls him, that no invisible walls exist. The patient must sincerely believe in his mind and feel in his heart that he does have a choice, that the real answers are within, that the right knowledge with action is the power. This may take time and patience. It is sad when a patient gives up with a feeling that destiny or fate is involved in creating the misfortune.

I have seen many clients whose parents died because of smoking. The client will come in telling me that he wants to stop smoking, but he does not believe that he can do so. He continues to tell everyone that his father died of smoking, and surely he will too. The identification is powerful. It is as if the patient wears a label on his forehead that says: "I am my father. I must die of smoking." Until that imaginary label is dispensed with, the client will smoke until he dies. Similarly, many other people literally hypnotize themselves unconsciously to believe that because a parent or a brother or a sister had a problem, they will have the same problem. However, constantly fearing the problem may make it happen.

When It Is Necessary to Dehypnotize

When a patient's mind already has been hypnotized with an idea, it is more expedient to dehypnotize him. Positive hypnotic suggestions can be given that he is one of a kind; a special individual; as unique as his fingerprints and voice prints; that he has had many experiences unlike his father; that he is not his father; that he can rip the label off and may keep the best of his father in his personality without smoking.

A large number of positive mental images may be projected onto his subconscious mind screen as he remains in hypnosis with his mind concentrated. These suggestions may involve seeing himself enjoying his new life as a nonsmoker. In hypnosis, an auditory hallucination may be induced so he hears his father's voice congratulating him on stopping smoking.

Some people place labels on themselves, like a label on a bottle. Because they believe the label strongly, all their actions lead them toward the maintenance of that thought. A life can be ruined by a bad label, such as "I am inadequate" or "I am poor at sports" or "I cannot control my temper." Identifying with a mother, a father, a brother, a sister, or a significant other strongly intensifies the negative labeling. However, strong identification with positive labels, such as "all my siblings are successful, so I can be successful too" may be most beneficial.

The Power of Belief

Here's an example of the power of belief and labeling. As a teenager, I met a young man named Cliff. He had been hypnotized before. When people learn how to be hypnotized, it is easier for them to do it again, because being hypnotized is a skill. Like playing a piano, typing, or riding a bicycle, we get better with practice.

Anyway, Cliff had a broken arm, which had been successfully treated by a physician. However, he was left with pain. He wanted me to hypnotize him to eliminate the pain. I pulled a bottle of pills from my pocket and asked him to "take just one because they are powerful hypnotic pills." I asked him to lie down on the couch and in about 10 seconds he was in hypnosis. In fact, in about five seconds, he was unable to stand up and he told me he had to lie down.

The amazing part of all this was that the prescription bottle, which I had labeled "Hypnotics" and shown to Cliff, contained placebos, pills that had no effect. I reinforced the message on the label with waking suggestions: "These pills are powerful." The process was complete. He already had given his permission to be hypnotized by asking for hypnosis. He was motivated to be hypnotized in order to eliminate his pain. Most importantly, his expectation of hypnosis was high.

The experiment was a success. The placebo worked and Cliff's pain left him following my hypnotic suggestion that his arm would feel a little numb and with no discomfort. This was a direct suggestion without any need for elaborate mental imagery using all the senses. Some clients need far more detailed imagery and training to dissolve the pain.

I also told Cliff while he was in hypnosis that this would be a temporary numbness. I did not want him to have a numb arm for the rest of his life. Also, if there was a medical problem, I wanted it to surface so he could see his physician.

The power of belief is most evident in the story of the prisoner who was to be executed by draining his blood. This individual lay on the table and the doctor feigned a small cut on his arm. Because there was no cut, there really was no blood loss. However, the sound of water dripping into a pail was heard. The prisoner, believing his blood was leaving him, died.

51

Don't Silence the Warning Signs

Too many people often forget that pain, headaches, stomach aches, heart palpitations, eye strain, and other symptoms normally are warning signals to change something in their lives. These symptoms are red flags saying: "Notice me. It's time to change your lifestyle or your attitudes." Even professional healers often do not do what they teach others. They don't listen to their bodies and instead allow themselves to be caught up in the treadmill of stress, poor diet, lack of exercise, lack of sleep, lack of a vacation, and overscheduling work.

When I was younger I was on a treadmill. I often worked more than 100 hours a week. One month I performed 28 shows in 28 cities and appeared at radio and television interviews at the same time. Time and the years go by rapidly when you are so busy. Every city became a blur. I felt life went by fast enough, and the travel and excessive work were speeding it up.

I traveled for several reasons. I enjoyed entertaining audiences and inspiring them with a thrilling performance. The hypnotic shows were a dramatic display of the possibilities of the human mind and the potential to overcome inhibition for change. Hypnosis released the creativity of a hypnotized volunteer so that he could easily do what he would have deemed impossible in the normal wide awake state. Shy, inhibited people became extroverts in minutes, even seconds. It's really amazing what we can do when we believe in our mind and in our heart that we can succeed.

Finding the Solution in Your Mind

To most North Americans, the more "medical looking" the suggestion, the more powerful it is. Research has shown that a pill may be effective, a needle is stronger yet, and surgery is stronger still. Each method represents an increasing intrusion into the body. My own physician, Dr. Robson, tells me there are people who are obsessed with the belief that only surgery can cure them.

Both hetero-hypnosis and self-hypnosis present a wonderful opportunity to use this marvelous gift of the Creator to climb inside our own subconscious. The subconscious may be asked not only the cause of the problem, but more importantly for the best solution. A solution that comes from the inner mind of the client is generally the most effective. Through hypnoanalysis, it is possible for the therapist to draw out solutions from the client's subconscious. Techniques such as word association, the use of the subconscious movement of a pendulum to answer questions, and dream analysis may be helpful.

This is likely to be more effective than direct hypnotic suggestions by the therapist. In the rare case that the client draws a blank on solutions, the therapist can give vague clues that might be followed, instead of actual solutions. For example "you might solve this problem by going around it to the left, to the right, underneath, remove it, over it, or some other direction."

Still more amazing is the opportunity to practice this solution technique without a therapist. I do it all the time. When you are in touch with your inner mind, when you honor and respect your inner mind, the answers are forthcoming. This is a bond of inner friendship and trust as with your closest friend, which the subconscious is. When answers do come from your subconscious, it is important to thank your inner mind during and/or at the end of the experience.

With practice, the voice of your inner mind will give you information and answers more rapidly. The process will seem most natural, which it is. This is somewhat similar to hunches or intuition. Also, if these subconscious messages are ignored, they will come less often. Honor your messages as gifts for which to be thankful and they will come to you in great abundance. A relaxed mental state and expectation of solutions are the keys for the success of using 100 percent of your brain power.

Alcohol and Hypnosis

Another school friend, Brian, was not as easy to hypnotize as Helmut. I tried to overcome Brian's unconscious resistance to hypnosis, but I was unable to break through his "mental wall" during three sessions. Then one night before I hypnotized him, he had a beer. In this session, he was effortlessly guided into a relaxing trance. It is a common saying among hypnotists that a little alcohol is a hypnotist in its own right and this was proven to me the night Brian finally, and quickly, went into hypnosis.

However, if a person drinks too much alcohol, this ruins the concentration required to enter the trance. I once asked a volunteer to look into my eyes to be hypnotized. He said I see four of them, which one? I knew he had too much to drink!

Houdini would never touch alcohol. He said that it would ruin his mental concentration and the hair trigger coordination necessary for his escapes, some of which were definitely dangerous. Most of his escapes were illusions by a master; however, when something did go wrong, they became literally death-defying. I drink alcohol, but very little.

My friends and I made old silent home movies that document my beginning years of practicing hypnotism. What fun we had when someone's feet would be stuck to the floor or their personality would change or perhaps a past life would be discovered. Believers and non-believers in past lives are both in abundance. Woody Allen once said: "I don't believe in an afterlife, although I am bringing an extra change of underwear just in case."

The Unexplained Powers of the Mind

On several occasions, I hypnotized Brian and showed him the back of a playing card while I memorized the face of the card. Then I asked Brian to close his eyes while I shuffled the card into the deck. Then I asked him to open his eyes and to find the card, just looking at the back of the cards. In every case, he found the correct card! No kidding! I thought maybe he was seeing something on the back of the card that I did not notice and that perhaps this helped him to locate the correct card. So, I used a new deck, and he still found the correct card! Without being superstitious and without believing that he had extra-sensory perception, I believe he had some type of highly acute powers of observation. There are many unexplained powers of the mind that are in operation once you believe that you possess them. Hypnosis helps you to use 100 percent of your brain power.

Research experiments have proven repeatedly that if a person focuses his mind (with hypnosis or creative visualization) to believe that he possesses superhuman strength, he will indeed perform with greater strength than is possible without the mind focusing. You may have heard rumors of mothers lifting an automobile off an injured child. These are not rumors. They are documented cases. However, it is not uncommon that after performing such a herculean task, the mother has physical injury.

My awareness of this incredible hypnotic talent proved useful on many occasions when I gave stage presentations. In my early years, I wore contact lenses. Sometimes a lens would become dry and pop out onto the stage floor. When that occurred, I would tell one of the hypnotized volunteers that he was a detective with acute powers of observation and that a small contact lens had been lost. I never worried about losing the lens, because the hypnotized volunteer always found the lens within seconds.

Audiences never knew that the volunteer was actually searching for a real lens. The audience thought that the hypnotized volunteer was finding an imaginary lens. I would slip to the side of the stage, cleanse the lens, and pop it into my eye. These heightened powers of observation shown by hypnotized people represent only one of many talents that are enhanced under hypnosis. Hypnotic suggestions may be given additional power if an imagined situation is created such as "your life or the life of your loved one depends upon your success."

What a drastic improvement my techniques have achieved since those early years. But when I look back, I was still pretty good. I remember numerous standing ovations from audiences. In essence, the hypnotist has to be a knowledgeable guide to draw out the best of that which resides within the hypnotized person's subconscious mind.

A large percentage of the population can actually enjoy a rapid entrance into hypnosis, even on the first experience. This could be as fast as seconds. When I was in my teens, twenties, and thirties, I presented theatrical hypnosis throughout the United States and Canada. It was easy to pick out the special folks on stage who had focused attention. The head was basically motionless, and the eyes were fixed in a gaze. The expression had to be serious. I would merely walk over to the person and say: "Focus on my right eye. Your eyes are growing heavy. Your arms are growing heavy. Your legs are growing heavy. Your entire body is growing heavy. Your eyes are heavy. Your arms are heavy. Your legs are heavy. Your entire body is heavy. Your eyes are closing, closing, closing, closing. Close your eyes and sleep."

If I noticed very strong concentration, I would just look at the person's eyes and shout "Sleep!" If I presented a concert of hypnotism to a larger audience, such as the Pacific National Exhibition in

Vancouver, Canada, the approach was slightly different. In an audience of 5,000 people, hundreds of people volunteered to be hypnotized on stage. Once the stage was full with about 200 volunteers, I would simply walk to the center of the stage, wave my hand, and just shout "Sleep!" This allowed me to move on with the show rapidly rather than spend a lot of time conducting a long tedious hypnotic induction. Sometimes, while facing the volunteers, I emphasized the suggestion by simultaneously closing my eyes and dropping my head down to my chest while I shouted the word "Sleep!"

These volunteers were eager to be hypnotized. Most had never been hypnotized before, yet we would always hypnotize many more than were needed. We would end up having to "awaken" many of the volunteers, because the stage would be too crowded for a fast moving show if we left everyone hypnotized.

The methods I used over a decade ago on stage are not really appropriate for clinical use. There are other more elegant methods to rapidly hypnotize first-timers and the more experienced. These methods are useful to speed up the hypnotizing process so that more time is left for the actual therapy.

Pacing and Leading

I remember hypnotizing a woman at a seminar in Massachusetts. I sat at a small table across from the woman and began to match my eye movements to hers. As we faced each other, if her eyes darted to her left, mine went to my right, and vice versa. After a moment or so of doing this, I judged she was about to be hypnotized rapidly, so I began moving my body to the left, right, up, and down in a similar way. Within a couple of minutes, she was following my movements. All I had to do was to begin acting as though my eyes were heavy and relaxed. I let my eyelids close and open slowly, several times. Within seconds, her eyes had closed and remained closed. She was in a state of hypnosis—without a word being spoken.

This is an example of the neurolinguistic programming (NLP) techniques of pacing and leading. The pacing refers to one doing what the other does until there is a rapport or "mental bonding." I "paced" when I kept up with her eye and body movements. When this mental connection was felt, I then "led" her. This was successful because there was an element of trust between the two of us. She was there because she wanted to be hypnotized.

When I gave lecture-demonstrations and theatrical performances to large groups, I would sometimes hypnotize the entire group
by mail or telegram. The participants would be seated in a large
semicircle facing the audience and I would give a card to someone
at the end of the semicircle. The card read as follows: "You are
getting very sleepy. Please hand this card to the next person. Close
your eyes and sleep." I have also hypnotized people on the telephone
for the elimination of various unhealthy habits. This could be done
by radio, television, or even skywriting with an airplane.

I should make it clear that hypnosis is not actually sleep. Hypnosis is an altered state of consciousness wherein one is actually
more awake than asleep. Many clients will be hypnotized and follow
all the hypnotic suggestions given to them, yet they may come out
of hypnosis saying: "I don't think I was hypnotized because I was
not asleep." This belief can ruin an otherwise beneficial hypnosis
session. The person can leave the session thinking, "I guess I was
not hypnotized. I sure don't feel like smoking. I don't want to have
a cigarette, but I don't think I was hypnotized. Maybe it didn't work.
I may as well have a cigarette since it probably didn't work." Some
clients will even force themselves to have a cigarette, to make a test
of the power of the hypnotist's work. The client literally can talk
himself out of the benefits he has received. It is a good idea to
convince the client that he was indeed hypnotized, before he leaves
the session.

Brain Power Techniques

In hypnosis, you feel very relaxed in body and mind. This is a
highly prized gift for use with today's stressful lifestyle. With the
consistent use of hypnosis, one can truly restore mental health,
physical health, energy, and a positive mental attitude. A simple
method is to just mentally relax parts of your body from the bottom
of your feet to the top of your head. Another simple method, which
can be combined with the above technique, is to focus upon your
breath. You may imagine your breath to be a relaxing color. Imagine
the air as it flows smoothly throughout your body, nourishing every
cell. Be aware of the rising and falling of the chest. Breathe in
through your nose and out through your mouth. Breathe slowly and
deeply in a way that is comfortable for you. I have found this
exercise to be most beneficial to me. To relax, I imagine the breath

as a soothing pink color; to energize myself, I imagine the breath as an orange color.

These brain power methods are easy to use. A small child may even benefit from them. I often imagine a favorite place such as a quiet beach in Hawaii or in the Carribean. I am alone. The sound of the waves can be heard rolling in and out. I imagine seeing the puffs of white clouds slowly float across the beautiful blue sky and meet the crystal clear blue horizon. The water is filled with tropical fish of brilliant colors. All is calm. All is relaxed. I see the endless white sand and perhaps another island in the distance. I feel the warm sand between my toes and on my back as I lie down. The sun is warm, but I am protected by sunscreen and the shade of palm trees. Some have coconuts; some do not. There are papaya trees, guava trees, mango trees, banana trees, and many large colorful flowers. The more senses that you use, the better.

You can create a scene from memory and imagine it to be exactly as you want it. Or you can create an imaginary place where you have never been before, perhaps in another country or even another galaxy. An imaginary scene may be more relaxing than a scene from true memory. An imaginary scene may be perfect.

From time to time, I feel a breeze on my body cooling me off—whenever I need it. An occasional fishing boat, cruise ship, or airplane may be seen or heard in the distance. Perhaps I imagine I go for a long walk or a jog on the beach to develop a tired feeling and then I fall asleep. I enjoy running my fingers over seashells while studying their unique patterns. Perhaps I save an unusual rock that looks like a pancake. I may focus again on enjoying a few deep breaths and tell myself to enjoy relaxing deeper and deeper, more and more with every breath…deeper and deeper relaxed with every wave. This may be an excellent experience for overcoming insomnia.

I breathe in through my nose and out through my mouth. I feel the air passing through my body. I imagine I am filling up a huge glass. If I filled up a huge glass with water, I would fill up the bottom first and then the middle and then the top. I would empty the glass from the top, middle, and then the bottom. Similarly, I imagine my body filling up with air at the bottom, middle, and top. Then I exhale from my mouth, emptying the top, middle, and bottom.

I can also enjoy the intoxicating scent of beautiful flowers or perhaps the clean fresh air of the ocean. This is easy if you are a lover of flowers like I am. I have a large number of rose bushes in my yard. Each bush is a different variety and a different aroma.

By the way, I highly recommend that if you have not already done so that you visit an aromatherapy store. You can experience sensations of alertness, relaxation, sensuality, concentration, and energy with the various fragrances. For example, vanilla, lily of the valley, and apple spice are natural stress reducers. Having stored experiences of the pleasures of floral scents in the memory bank of your mind, you can use these in hypnosis. Just remembering the scents can recreate all the pleasures within you all over again.

You can even imagine having a cool, tall glass of your favorite drink. Be sure to add lots of ice cubes, perhaps a lemon or lime twist, or a cherry. These methods are fun to play with. Yes, they are an excursion into an altered state of consciousness. I call them a vacation without the cost of a ticket.

When you are in this altered mental state, pain may vanish like magic or at least diminish and teeth can be extracted without awareness. Thousands of surgical operations already have been carried out worldwide with just hypnosis as the sole anesthetic. Hypnosis also has been popular on the battlefield where it was used because it was the only anesthetic tool available. There is no more natural method than hypnosis, a gift from the Creator.

There Are No Zombies Here

Hypnosis is simply focused mental concentration on a single thought or idea. This mental focusing is induced by salespeople, ministers, nurses, physicians, teachers, parents, actors, and politicians. Whenever the goal is to focus our attention upon accepting someone else's ideas, principles of hypnotism are in use.

I cannot overemphasize that you are not asleep when you are in hypnosis. Hypnosis has long been connected with sleep because of the early belief that hypnosis was sleep. About 1841, Scottish physician James Braid coined the terms "hypnotism" and "hypnosis" from the Greek word "hypnos," which means sleep. Braid later realized that hypnosis is not sleep, but the term already had gained widespread acceptance. Similarly, you do not really "awaken" from hypnosis. You *come out* of hypnosis.

Today, fiction books, movies, and television shows continue to portray hypnosis as a strange sleep-like condition wherein one is a zombie under someone's control. Strange connections of hypnosis to the supernatural, astrology, numerology, fortune-telling, and other allied arts is still seen today. With this book, I hope to clarify many misconceptions about hypnosis.

However, as with all professions, the instructors need proper training. One unqualified instructor easily leaves a black mark on the profession. If you only "think" a hypnotist is a hypnotist, please think again. Their skills vary greatly.

When people have difficulty using the techniques, it is often because they need a live professional instructor rather than a book or recordings. Or, an instructor with more varied techniques in his toolbox may be more successful. In this way, the techniques can be adapted to the individual personality of the client. Sometimes hypnosis does not work simply because the client does not personally like that hypnotist. Perhaps they would feel more comfortable with the same sex, opposite sex, a smaller person, a different manner, or a hypnotist with a different appearance. Perhaps that hypnotist reminds them of someone they do or don't like.

Sometimes people give up on hypnosis when it does not work right away. However, often permanent changes take time and repeated re-hypnotizing. That's why hypnotic recordings, which provide repetition and reinforcement of suggestions, are valuable.

Hypnosis does not create "zombies." Even under the deepest hypnosis, there is an awareness of the surroundings. There is also what I call the *subconscious censor*, which protects us. For purposes of experimentation, I have asked people to reveal personal secrets before an audience of witnesses. I knew no personal secrets would be revealed. Actually, people are able to lie far better when hypnotized than when they are wide awake. This is because hypnotized people are more relaxed and, therefore, more creative. They can come up with all kinds of stories. If we did a past lives presentation, wherein people relive past lives, it was not unusual to have two or three Joan of Arcs the same week. People were more likely to recall being a famous person in a past life than being someone who scrubbed floors.

However, this does not negate the value of past lives therapy. If the client believes his past life is responsible for a problem in his present life, then this is true for him. An example is the case of the man who had constant headaches. He was hypnotized and revealed a past life wherein he was on top of a castle wall with a spear stuck in his head. In the past life, he fell in the moat below and died in the water. Under hypnosis, he was told: "This happened in a past life, in another body. That body is gone. You are in a new body. Everything is fine. You are okay." The man's headaches disappeared, never to return again.

By the time I was in my mid-teens, I was seriously interested in the therapeutic applications of hypnosis. Unfortunately, audiences were cautious of hypnotists and were more interested in them as entertainers than serious hypnotherapists. I presented my first hypnotic stage show to a large audience when I was 15. Looking back, it sounds like the script from a Hollywood film about a poor kid doing his shows to put food in his stomach.

I literally did shows in restaurants, like Dimitri's in Winnipeg, for a steak dinner. My first professional show paid me $60 for 20 minutes in front of a Christmas party of 800 people at the Marlborough Hotel in Winnipeg. That was a lot of money then, but I did not do hypnosis to make a lot of money. I did it because I found it fascinating. I was booked by a local agent and entertainer named Len Andree of Andree Productions. He watched my early performances, in which I spent most of the performance staring at the ceiling, and advised me to improve my showmanship. I was able to rapidly hypnotize a number of people, but, Len said, I didn't know what to do with them after I hypnotized them.

And so, I began studying the art of public speaking and showmanship. I believe public speaking is one of the best skills a person can learn. Being able to speak easily and well in front of others boosts confidence. Great communication skills go a long way toward helping a person to be successful in both the business and social arena. I'm happy and proud that my older daughter Diana joined the public speaking club at her high school. Surprisingly, few students have indicated an interest in joining the club. Diana's public speaking skills are certainly better than mine were when I was her age.

If you have been using negative self-talk or negative self-imagery before you make a speech in public, you probably are not presenting up to your potential. With brain power methods, you can visualize a positive reaction to your speaking. You can make a hypnosis cassette tape with suggestions and imagery for a confident and competent speaking presentation. The use of recordings is most beneficial because they help to focus your attention and intensify your concentration, which is fundamental to the efficient use of hypnosis. After using recordings for a few weeks, you probably will find that you can induce an effective brain power mental state even without a recording.

To further my career in hypnosis, in my late teens, I decided to contact an internationally known magician in Calgary, Micky Hades. Micky gave me valuable instruction in the areas of stage hypnosis, mentalism, and showmanship. Mentalism is the art of mental magic for entertainment and includes predictions, mind-reading, and psychometry. The Amazing Kreskin is perhaps the most recognized entertainer in the area of mental magic. Micky's advice filled me with energy and confidence for my future performances. Countless other entertainers, psychologists, physicians, hypnotists, and business people have been willing to share their knowledge with me over the years. For this, I am very grateful.

Throughout those early years I collected books on everything having to do with wellness, psychology, hypnosis, mental magic, public speaking, humor, and presentation skills. On the business side, I accumulated a large amount of information dealing with advertising, publicity, general promotion, marketing, and financial survival. I sought information through personal contacts, books, and seminars. The books I could not buy, I borrowed from the library for months on end. However, the real magic of theatrical hypnosis is in the showmanship, the make-up, the dress, the tone of voice, the performer's stories connected to the effect, the confidence of the presenter, as well as his sense of humor. After all, the number one goal is to be entertaining.

Many years ago, I drove from Winnipeg to Milwaukee, Wisconsin, to see a show by a well-loved U.S. hypnotist and ESP entertainer, Gil Eagles. The next morning we had breakfast together, and Gil was kind enough to share many of his professional secrets. Gil told me to look at the phrase "show business." He said, "Notice which word is longer and the most important." Indeed, without employing the skills of a businessman, the hypnotist is soon out of business. He can help no one when he is bankrupt, starving, and his number one concern is looking for food.

Theatrical Hypnosis

Throughout my years of touring as an entertainer, there was a small group in the medical community who declared that hypnosis on stage was inappropriate. Theatrical hypnosis was considered as inappropriate as allowing the public to watch a surgical operation. Today I can observe detailed surgical procedures from my living room sofa. Recently I watched a television program showing doctors performing a vasectomy and a tubal ligation—the latter with hypnosis as the only anesthetic. It was all in living color and blasted across my 45-inch screen.

Actually, it was the stage hypnotists who helped keep interest in hypnosis alive. By exposing the methods to millions of people, interest was generated in the clinical possibilities. However, I must admit that, like every profession, a few bad apples can make the entire profession appear unfavorable. A truly great concert hypnotist makes sure his volunteers leave the stage feeling alert, refreshed, and full of energy as though they have been on a long vacation. He removes all the theatrical suggestions of personality changes.

The volunteer should leave the stage feeling fantastic and extremely confident because mental blocks and inhibitions have been removed. These good feelings, without any further reinforcement, can last for weeks, months, and even years.

There have been some hypnotists who have used hypnosis for vulgar presentations in some night clubs, billing themselves perhaps as x-rated. Sometimes night club volunteers may be less inhibited by the alcohol than by the hypnosis. Indeed, if the hypnotist asks them to do something in the way of exhibitionism, they may welcome the opportunity. In other words, at last they can do whatever they have always wanted to do, however outrageous, and get away with it by blaming the hypnotist!

They make the hypnotist the scapegoat saying: "He made me do it; I couldn't help it." Or, "That's ridiculous! I never did that." They may need denial to save face or true amnesia of the event.

Unfortunately, the obscene usually is more profitable. For example, the film *Sliver* had weak box office sales in North America.

Paramount decided to insert a few minutes of steamy sexual content for the overseas version. The advertising proclaimed: "The picture America didn't see." The overseas ticket sales were double the North American sales.

When I gave presentations in schools and colleges, I often ended the presentation with "brain power gifts." The sponsor, often a principal or entertainment coordinator, might ask me to give the students hypnotic suggestions for improvements in sports, concentration, memory, help with being relaxed during exams, or perhaps help to eliminate smoking or overeating.

Even in the 1960s, I was interested in applying hypnosis to smoking cessation and weight control. My mother, who wanted to maintain her weight, regularly exercised in front of our black and white RCA television. At that time, my father had a serious bout with a pre-cancerous warning on one of his lips due to his smoking. He contracted leukoplakia meaning white patch. Doctors call this "smoker's patch." One in 20 cases of leukoplakia eventually will become malignant and may fatally spread throughout the mouth and throat. Leukoplakia of the larynx or voice box of a smoker is responsible for the raspy, gravel voice so commonly associated with smoking.

Our family was concerned about my father's health. His lip was surgically cut and cleansed of the malignant tissue. This left a deep impression on me, and I felt even stronger about pursuing hypnosis to help people overcome their habits. My father quit smoking immediately when he was told about the problem, but fear of disease and death does not always help someone to stop smoking.

In August 1994, researchers told a panel of the U.S. Food and Drug Administration that about 40 per cent of people who have their larynxes removed because of smoking promptly resume smoking cigarettes, using the hole in their necks to inhale. I have a sign on my file cabinet that says: "Cancer cures smoking." Unfortunately, there are people who really believe in their heart that they cannot change; that because a parent died from smoking, they must too; or that life is just not worth living and they hope to die young. To this latter group, cigarettes are just another form of slow motion suicide, a somewhat personally and socially acceptable way to kill oneself. After all, they can say, "I didn't kill myself; the cigarettes did."

Success Principles

As a young child, I was greatly influenced by my mother for she introduced me to positive thinking and setting goals for a successful life. I remember a daily routine of sitting with her at breakfast and listening to Earl Nightingale's inspirational radio programs. His enthusiastic professional broadcaster voice and his great stories, each of which taught a lesson on successful living, were broadcast on hundreds of radio stations in North America. My mother and I discussed each radio broadcast. His magical messages helped me to realize that there are specific important success principles. These principles can be learned to help one overcome negativity, and having goals is one of the most important.

In eighth grade, Mr. A. Bryant, the instructor of my guidance and counseling class at Churchill High School, played Earl Nightingale's famous record, *The Strangest Secret*. This record re-affirmed my belief that whatever we think about the most, we become. We can completely change our life by setting goals and by changing our thoughts. Here are a few of my favorite quotations on the subject:

- "All that we are is the result of what we have thought. The mind is everything. What we think, we become."—Buddha
- "The happiness of your life depends upon the quality of your thoughts, therefore guard accordingly; and take care that you entertain no notions unsuitable to virtue and reasonable nature."—Marcus Antoninus
- "Great men are they who see that spiritual is stronger than any material force—that thoughts rule the world."—Ralph Waldo Emerson
- "Whatever the mind of man can conceive and believe, the mind of man can achieve."—Napoleon Hill
- "Imagination rules the world." —Napoleon Bonaparte
- "Most folks are about as happy as they make their minds to be."—Abraham Lincoln

A few years ago, after having admired Earl Nightingale's radio show, recordings, and books for many years, I had the wonderful opportunity to hear Earl Nightingale speak to a large audience in Vancouver, British Columbia. For me, this was a highlight in my life. Unfortunately, Earl died shortly thereafter. His company Nightingale Conant continues today in Chicago, Illinois, as the world's largest distributor of self-improvement and motivational recordings for personal and corporate use.

The *Bible* proclaims, "If thou canst believe, all things are possible." My father always told me, "You make your own luck." On the other hand, if we do not have goals, we will achieve nothing. When events went awry in my life as a young man, my father would look at me and with his wry sense of humor say: "Life is grim." Dad had a way of making me smile every time he said that.

Often when I do hypnosis with a group, I will from time to time whisper hypnotic suggestions over and over such as: "You really are fantastic. You really are fantastic. You really are fantastic." The repetition increases the power of the suggestion. Because of the altered state of consciousness, the mind is susceptible to absorbing these positive suggestions for belief in one's own capacities and skills. People will tell me that it feels wonderful to hear positive suggestions repeated in hypnosis, because most of their life they have been ignored or, when spoken to, mostly only with negative suggestions.

I also can thank my mother for teaching me many other aspects of life such as ethics, morals, fairness, and the sanctity of one's good reputation. I was always taught to be fair. Giving someone their money's worth was just as important as being successful. I have always given my all when doing shows, seminars, private sessions, or recordings.

Hypnotizing others often requires a great deal of concentration on the part of the hypnotist. Because of the focused attention given by the hypnotist, the use of the technique can sometimes be emotionally draining for the hypnotist. The work rapidly can lead to exhaustion and burnout. I used to experience this, but now I make sure there are points during the hypnosis session when I give a positive suggestion to the client, I also imagine that the same suggestion is simultaneously being given to me.

After being a laborer for many years, my father decided to open his own business. My mother feared he would go bankrupt, but my father convinced her that he knew what he was doing, and he did! Shortly after he started the business, his brother Neno, who was also a railroad employee, became his partner. Within two years, they had built a successful business selling automobile parts. Dad was happy.

He was doing what he liked to do and making money at it. That was success. He satisfied people's wants and they rewarded him with adequate prosperity.

We were still far from being rich, but we had all that we needed and we were happy. If we look around today, we see that low-income earners are still living the life of kings and queens, compared to millions of people suffering poverty in other countries. How often is someone unhappy because they want far more than they really need?

I have been in communication via email with a woman in Hawaii named Linda. She had an automobile accident at age 15. Her left ankle was crushed. For 25 years she has had chronic pain and mobility problems. As she says: "There are some things that people, or most people take for granted, like the ability to walk anywhere. Physical pain is far worse than emotional pain."

As I tell you about Linda in Hawaii, I am reminded of perhaps the strangest experience that I have ever had. In the early 70s, I dated a young woman in Winnipeg named Lynn. Eventually, we drifted apart and stopped dating. A few months after we stopped seeing each other, my brother Dave and I went on a two-week vacation to Honolulu. During the trip, Dave came down with a cold and spent most of the time in bed at the Pacific Beach Hotel.

One day I went to the beach alone and, as I sunbathed in the warm sand, I wished Lynn was there with me. About 10 minutes later, I looked up and I thought I saw Lynn wearing a sun hat, sitting on the sand about 30 feet from me. The woman sure looked like Lynn, except she had a different hairstyle and a young man was sitting beside her.

About two years later, I visited Lynn and she showed me photos of herself in Hawaii. You guessed it! Lynn had been on that beach wearing a sun hat. Could this be a coincidence that I would focus upon the one person in more than 4 billion and that that person would appear in front of me? Or could this be a strange form of psychic mind power? Unlikely as it may seem, I think the former is probably true, but you never know. If you have had a similar experience, please share it with me by writing to: Vance Romane, Box 75177, White Rock, British Columbia, Canada V4A 9N4. I may include your experience in my next book.

6

Financial Stress

I know of a famous rock star who had a home in the state of Washington with 28 bedrooms, an indoor pool, five acres, plus a separate building housing a recording studio. I was told by a real estate agent that, although the entertainer could have afforded to keep the house, he let it go into foreclosure where it sold for a fraction of the value. Apparently, the rock star had simply said that kind of lifestyle was no longer for him.

Mother Teresa once arrived to open a new mission. Nice new carpets were placed on the floor of the building. On arrival, she had the carpets ripped off the floor and thrown outside. She did not want to display a better lifestyle than is experienced by those whom she helps. Mother Teresa, the Roman Catholic nun who has devoted her life to India's poor, was awarded the Nobel Peace Prize in 1979. At the award ceremony in Oslo, the chairman of the committee, Professor John Sanness, said Mother Teresa deserved the prize "because she promotes peace in the most fundamental manner—by her confirmation of human dignity." Mother Teresa asked that the traditional peace-prize dinner be canceled so that its cost of $6,000 could be used to assist in her work. There is a growing trend to stop trying to accumulate so many material goods, to choose a simpler life.

I have found that the larger a home someone buys, the more "stuff" they tend to accumulate, most of which is not necessary. My father taught me to ask myself one simple question before I buy something: "Do you really need it?" His father always told him: "Easy to buy, hard to sell." My father also told me to earn enough money to feel free to do what I want to do. Money does buy freedom to pursue life as you wish. I make sacrifices so my family can enjoy a reasonably good standard of living. However, there is a limit to how much money I really need. Life is short and time to pursue my own interests and those in the best interest of my family take precedence over stockpiling more money than I need.

A friend who was about 30 years older than I once asked me if I would trade ages for his savings (over $17 million) and I had to say no. I know he would gladly trade all his money for youth and health. Problems with hearing, sight, and other ailments are all too common with age. Aunt Grace, who has a great sense of humor, once said: "Every morning I wake up, I know I'll have a pain, but I don't know where it will be."

If you make up your mind, you can live for less. I have traveled to many places, and I have investigated real estate worldwide on the Internet. I have found that where you may buy a beautiful home in a big city for a million dollars or a half million dollars, you can buy the same beautiful home in a relaxing rural community in another state or province for up to 90 percent less.

Today many businesses can be conducted anywhere with computers, modems, and fax machines. If one wishes to leave the cold for a month or two in the winter, there are ways to travel that are less expensive, yet more fun. For example, you may be able to negotiate with a bed and breakfast operator for an economical, lengthy, off-season visit. Some may even exchange homes to go to a cold, inhospitable climate simply because they have never seen snow before. There are thousands of bed and breakfast operators and worldwide home exchange organizations listed in your local library.

Recently, a money management consultant told me corporations are requesting fewer stress reduction seminars and more money management seminars. Apparently, many corporations have found that most of the stress occurring today in people's lives comes from financial stress. His seminar teaches employees how to handle money better, how to save, and how to invest. His clients appreciate the stress reduction in their employees, and there is less need for advancing wages to employees or increasing wages.

Lack of money has become a major problem for many people and could get far worse with layoffs, increasing government taxes, and perhaps a sudden change in interest rates. You have more control over your life if you run your own business. If you are lucky enough to reach 65, the traditional age of retirement, your chance of being able to sustain the lifestyle you've grown accustomed to is only about 16 percent—that's not high.

The Importance of Education

My father only finished sixth grade, and my mother did not have an opportunity to finish high school when she was young. However, my father became a successful business owner and my mother completed her Bachelor of Arts Degree at the University of Manitoba— long after her children were grown. My parents gave me the courage to pursue my own dreams.

When I was performing in my teens, a local promoter named Henry Koopmans approached me about touring a number of fine concert halls in Canada, starting in the Okanagan Valley in British Columbia during the busy tourist season. My mother and I took the promoter's contract to a lawyer. The lawyer advised me to continue my schooling instead going on tour. I did so with a sense of disappointment then, but also with the understanding that education was a more important goal at that time of my life.

A few days later I went to a crowded discotheque called The Pink Panther. A young man approached me and asked if I would help him to stop smoking. He had recognized me from a performance at a charity function, and he was willing to be hypnotized on the spot. Within 30 seconds, he had entered a deep trance.

I had always read that hypnosis is best done in a quiet, secluded place with no distractions. This theory was proved false when I hypnotized him in the middle of the dance floor with the music and the crowd surrounding us. The loud speakers were 20 feet away and blaring "Shakin' All Over." I don't think anyone in the audience even knew that I had just hypnotized someone. Four years later, the man was still a nonsmoker.

After I graduated from high school, I enrolled in the psychology program at the University of Manitoba. During my first year at college, at age 18, I advertised a weekend seminar in hypnosis. I wanted to share my discoveries of how hypnosis can improve the quality of life. I still have old reel to reel tapes of that first brain power training program in 1967.

Looking back, I'm amazed that I had so much to talk about in those days. The attention span of people was longer in those days, too. Today, most people want to completely change everything in an evening and, for many people, that is too long. When I gave theatrical hypnosis concerts in the '60s, an audience easily could be entertained non-stop for three hours. Today, audiences are often happy with a 60-minute evening concert.

Back to the weekend seminar, only 13 people attended, but everyone learned a great deal about the mind. The group learned how hypnosis worked, how to hypnotize themselves, and how to apply it in their life in a multitude of areas. I really enjoyed giving the program, and I was pleased to see them all leave satisfied with what I had taught them. I continued to study hypnosis, and I had the opportunity to take seminars to improve my own skills. I found all of my university courses interesting, but often they covered a lot of material that was already familiar to me.

I began to feel the need to learn more about hypnosis and not just rehash all the techniques used by most fledgling hypnotists. In those days, I was the only hypnotist listed in the telephone book. Not only were there a limited number of hypnotists in North America, but there were a limited number of books and professional journal articles on the subject of hypnosis. Today there are thousands of hypnotists and thousands of physicians and psychologists who use hypnosis. The library of printed, audio, and video material on the subject is so large no one could possibly read everything that is published. The rapid growth in the profession alone attests to its acceptance as a valuable method of healing. Yet, this is a gift everyone should use—on a daily basis.

I wasn't in college long before I began to feel pressure from my professors. I didn't approach hypnosis—or even psychology—by the book and that disturbed them. It seemed to me that most of my professors were locked into the rigid thinking of the time. To me, they were like the false prophets of the past:

1902—"Flight by machines heavier than air is impractical and insignificant, if not utterly impossible."—Astronomer Simon Newcomb

1913—"It is an idle dream to imagine that ... automobiles will take the place of railways."—American Road Congress

1927—"Who the hell wants to hear actors talk?"—Harry Warner of Warner Brothers Studios

1977—"There is no reason for any individual to have a computer in their home."—Ken Olsen, president of Digital Equipment Corporation

Caleb C. Colton once stated: "The greatest friend of truth is time; her greatest enemy is prejudice..." An unknown author writes: "All truth passes through three stages: first it is ridiculed; next it is violently opposed; third it is accepted as being self-evident." In 1969, I attended a two-and-one-half-day course in Scientific Hypnotism and Self-Hypnosis conducted by Maurice Kershaw of the Canadian Institute of Hypnotism in Montreal. This was an excellent workshop. Many different types of people attended, including physicians. I sat next to one physician and tried to discuss hypnosis with him. However, the conversation rapidly came to a close when I mentioned I had hypnotized a number of people. In the fifties and sixties, many physicians and psychologists would not even admit to their colleagues that they had been to a hypnosis workshop. Hypnosis was associated with black magic, fortune-telling, and witchcraft.

In my opinion, the field of psychology can be a closed profession. Some associations have rules that members are not to associate with or share information with anyone who does not have a doctorate or at least a master's degree. I have had clinical psychologists tell me that they "shouldn't even be talking to" me. Dr. William J. Bryan, Jr., M.D., believed everyone should be allowed to take his hypnosis courses, because "education should never be denied anyone." I am of the same opinion; however, the ethics and morals of the student should be a major concern.

I attended the university for four years. During my last three years, I chose exclusively courses in psychology and sociology. I completed courses such as Criminology, Social Psychology, Developmental Psychology, Normal and Abnormal Psychology, Social Problems, Motivation, History of Psychology, Experimental Child Psychology, Medical Sociology, Physiological Psychology, Research Methods, Psychological Tests, Psychotherapy, and several courses in psychological research that were mandatory. However, my main interest was clinical psychology, not research.

Ever since childhood, I have wanted to help others to be happier, to enjoy life more. Generally, my interests have always been in the area of helping people with common everyday problems. This includes helping people to conquer smoking, achieve weight control, build self-esteem, or overcome stress, fears, guilt, obsessions, and compulsions. I also am interested in teaching people how to use self-induced relaxation, positive affirmations, and creative visualization. Brain power training helps people to feel empowered, to achieve their personal best, and even to become financially independent in a career of their choice.

My area of interest and expertise has not been to help people with psychotic reactions, wherein there is considerable lost contact with reality. These are more serious problems best helped by a clinical psychologist or a psychiatrist.

In the 1960s and early 1970s, most therapists had little knowledge or exposure to the field of hypnosis. Because they did not understand it, they did not accept it. Strange as it seems, all of their intensive therapeutic interviews had to involve mind focusing, direct and indirect suggestion, altered states of consciousness, and trances. Many therapists use hypnosis with their clients without realizing they are doing so.

During my fourth year at the university, I had to complete what was called a pre-master's thesis, a small research project. I decided to compare the effectiveness of hypnosis as compared to non-hypnosis methods to help people stop smoking. Dr. Morgan Wright, a clinical psychologist in the department, offered to oversee my project. In his words, "I really do not know much about hypnosis, but I'd like to do it with you." He had an attitude of let's do this together and we can both learn something. He was also my professor for Normal and Abnormal Psychology and my favorite professor.

During my entire university education, I only had one short class which discussed hypnosis and that was taught by Dr. Wright. Like many universities, my undergraduate program of psychology emphasized research, particularly experiments with rats. People were of more interest to me than rats. Still, I agreed with my professors that an understanding of research methodology was important so that I could better judge the results. However, it is also true that some research is not only bungled research, but purposely manipulated to show the results desired to continue obtaining grants or just to make less work for the researcher. Don't believe everything you read in research results.

As a matter of fact, one student told me that he carefully designed his research project and used imaginary statistics to tabulate his results. His professors believed that he had used real volunteers, and he laughed that he had fooled them. There were no real volunteers. The student is now a practicing psychologist with a doctorate in psychology.

The main reason I enrolled in the undergraduate psychology program was because of my interest in hypnosis. My four years at university provided a good education and valuable exposure to journal research. I am glad I was introduced to the work of such well respected names as Dr. Albert Ellis, Dr. Carl Rogers, Dr. Rollo May, Dr. Joseph Wolpe, Dr. Sidney M. Jourard, Dr. Andrew Salter, and many others. Their techniques helped me refine my hypnosis skills. There is no question that a background in psychology is important for an understanding of the mind and hypnosis. Learning the vocabulary of psychology and other health professions is absolutely essential to understanding and using hypnosis effectively.

Today, reading is my favorite pastime. I have thousands of books, audio cassettes, and videotapes. For a few dollars, I can climb inside someone's mind and learn something fascinating. I am never bored. There is always so much to read, so many people to talk to, and so much to do in exploring this wonderful world around us.

Over the years I have enjoyed programs with: Associate Trainers in Clinical Hypnosis; Dr. Elisabeth Kubler-Ross; Dr. Virginia Satir; David Calof and Steven Feldman, hypnotherapy training; Dr. Stephen Gillgan and Dr. Paul Carter, Intensive in Ericksonian Hypnotherapy; Institute of Applied Hypnology; Louise Hay; Dr. Deepak Chopra; Dr. Joan Borysenko; Shakti Gawain; The Academy For Guided Imagery with Dr. David Bresler and Dr. Martin Rossman; Ormond McGill; the Canadian Institute of Hypnotism with Maurice Kershaw; Dr. Joseph Barber, Hypnosis in Pain Control; Dr. Freda Morris, Hypnotherapy Training; Dr. Howard Eisenberg; Frank Stoss, M.D., and Anne Linden, Neuro-Linguistic Programming; and many workshops on stress control including an unforgettable lecture by Dr. Hans Selye. Dr. Selye gave a dramatic film presentation of the havoc stress contributes to the destruction of the body. When I attended the "Hypnotist Training Program" by Dr. Freda Morris, she told me that she had never had a student who knew as much about hypnosis as I did.

Additional seminars I have enjoyed covered such topics as medical, dental and legal hypnosis; the treatment of sexual disorders; man's search for happiness; and hypnoanalysis. I have also enjoyed numerous hypnosis conventions. Each year, more than 1,500 hypnotists attend the National Guild of Hypnotists Convention in Nashua, New Hampshire. There, one has the opportunity to attend lectures by dozens of colleagues, choosing from more than 200 workshops. There are many other conventions as well such as the Gil Boyne Annual Hypnotherapy Conference in Los Angeles, the Ericksonian Hypnotherapy Conference in Phoenix, the Society of Clinical and Experimental Hypnosis, and the International Medical and Dental Hypnotherapy Association in Royal Oak, Michigan.

Attendees at conventions range from doctors and nurses to ministers and police officers. Because hypnosis may be applied in every aspect of life, there is a diverse assortment of people who are interested in these techniques. Some conventions of psychologists, medical doctors, and psychiatrists will not permit anyone who does not have an advanced degree to attend, regardless of their knowledge of hypnosis. If you are not a member of their club, you may be excluded. At one time or another, medical doctors have wanted a hypnosis monopoly, as well as dentists and psychologists. Peter Reveen used to say that they just wanted to protect their own turf.

Exhibits of tapes, books, and various inventions that assist in the utilization of hypnotherapy are all on display at these conventions. The exchange of information and ideas with others in the profession is most enlightening because the convention participants come from all over the world.

After graduating from the university in 1971, I worked for a few months at The Canadian National Institute for the Blind. When my position at CNIB was eliminated, I was hired on at the Psychiatric Institute in Winnipeg. I worked under a clinical psychologist named Dr. Ivan Bilash. Dr. Bilash was a fine man who helped me increase my understanding about the mind and clinical psychology. He gave me instruction in Dr. Edmond Jacobson's relaxation therapy and psychological testing in areas such as intelligence, vocational, and personality testing. Although I was working with patients, I was not a "psychologist." When I gave a written evaluation of a patient, I was instructed to sign the form with my name and title, which was psychological technician.

Dr. Bilash was unpretentious, open, and receptive to my interest in hypnosis plus he wanted to use this remarkable tool in his psychotherapy practice. I shared some of my ideas and techniques with him when his patients needed help to stop smoking. He was always encouraging: "You'll find your niche." And he was right.

Dr. Bilash was open-minded toward procedures that were seldom practiced then, but which today are widely accepted. I admire people who are willing to jump out of the frame and try something new.

In late 1971, I finally realized that although I had been working part-time with hypnosis for a number of years, I wanted to work with hypnosis full time and independently on my own. Money was unimportant. I just wanted to pursue my fascination with the study of brain power skills to help others.

Taking the Show on the Road

At that time there was practically no demand for serious hypnotists, so I decided to increase my presence in the theatrical realm. I found it difficult to sell shows for a guaranteed fee, so I contracted engagements on percentages. When no guarantee was involved, the number of bookings I received increased dramatically. I obtained a number of contracts with 60 percent of the gate going to me. Frank Weipert, a University of Manitoba entertainment programmer, gave me the percentage idea. Frank was involved in bringing major acts to the university and also booked my show many times.

I soon gathered a large pile of testimonial letters from satisfied entertainment buyers. With established credibility, I was then able to increase my percentage to 80 percent and sometimes 90 percent. Unfortunately, sometimes 90 percent of next to nothing was about the same as nothing. Sometimes a sponsor booked the show, not to make a profit for his organization, but because he alone was personally interested in hypnosis. With little or no promotion from such an individual, there was no audience.

One night I was performing in a small city in British Columbia in the local auditorium. The performance was sponsored by a local school for entertainment value and to raise funds for their worthwhile projects. I had a full house, but few profits. Apparently, the teacher in charge of the receipts was intoxicated and left the cash boxes at the door while he enjoyed the show. When I mentioned we had a full house, he pointed to the cash box and said "that's all there is."

Although the bookings increased and I was able to make a modest living, it was difficult getting started. I was just a beginner in entertainment promotion. I can still remember one of my first direct mail campaigns. I sat in a cramped studio apartment in Regency Towers in Winnipeg and personally inserted, sealed, and stamped thousands of letters. In those days, stamps were just a few cents and I would send up to 5,500 in one mailing. On one rainy day, while carrying a large sack full of envelopes to the post office, the bag burst. Envelopes blanketed the sidewalk. Thankfully, Winnipeg was not as windy as usual on that embarrassing day.

I wrote to schools, halls, clubs, associations, colleges, entertainment agents, promoters, night clubs, fairs, exhibitions, and corporations throughout Manitoba. Len Andree, well known local entertainment agent, encouraged me to go nationally and, with his encouragement, I started to believe that if Manitoba accepted my shows so would other provinces.

During the next decade, I toured both Western and Eastern Canada as well as the United States. I toured as far west as Hawaii and as far east as Boston and Newfoundland. I also toured the Northwest and Yukon Territories. During those years, I enjoyed traveling and being on the road as a change of pace from private one-on-one hypnosis.

My most memorable show of the 1970s was at the Centennial Concert Hall in Winnipeg where I was billed at the "World's Fastest Hypnotist." Although this statement may have been correct, I am not sure it was to my benefit. I mass hypnotized more than 60 people in a matter of seconds, but later I discovered I hypnotized them too rapidly.

The ticket seller informed me after the show that some of those who witnessed my mass hypnotism did not believe it could be done as fast as I accomplished the feat. Some audience members assumed that I had used plants in the audience. I can say that I never have and

I never will use what in the trade is known as "confederates," "shills," "plants," or paid actors. Quite simply, it is not necessary; a public show always has plenty of willing people who are easily able to go into hypnosis. In the 1940s a hypnotist named Bob Nelson actually carried 20 paid actors. They would all act as if they were hypnotized. On one occasion, Bob was booked into a city where the folks quite simply were a different color. Using the plants was impossible, so Bob gave them all the day off. The show was great! He presented the same show as usual and hypnotized a large number of people from the audience. As a matter of fact, the show was better than ever because people on the stage were known to members of the audience. People love to see their friends hypnotized! As a result Bob fired all his plants, lowered his overhead, and had a more sensational show than ever! Plants are just not necessary, because hypnosis is a normal condition of everyday life, similar to daydreaming.

Using Imagery to Alter Consciousness

Hypnosis is a level of consciousness that is being neither awake nor asleep. Hypnosis is a state of heightened suggestibility normally characterized by focused or concentrated attention and often bodily relaxation. Music, focusing on deep breathing, isolation tanks, meditation, focusing upon a word such as "calm" over and over, running, massage, saunas, even warm baths can alter consciousness.

Any atmosphere that encourages imagery can alter consciousness. This may include:
- The scent of burning incense
- Lighting effects with flickering candles in darkness, stained glass windows
- Emotion-arousing music, repetitive sounds, chanting
- Symbolism with specific architectural designs, decor with pictures and ornate carvings, robes, etc.
- Point of fixation such as an altar, picture, candle flame, or cross
- Ceremony with certain rituals
- Sermon with repetitive ideas or sounds and specific voice inflections
- Silent meditation with eyes closed, focusing attention away from the outer world to the inner world of the mind
Any and all of these factors may aid the creation of an altered

state of consciousness, which some people call the superconscious state or a "higher self" state. The unfortunate fact is that this state also is capitalized on by more than 5,000 cults in America, which exploit followers under the guise of healing, personal growth, and self-actualization.

My most memorable show of the eighties was at the Pacific National Exhibition (PNE) in Vancouver, British Columbia. We held 33 evening concerts in 17 days. More than 50,000 people saw our presentations with up to 5,000 spectators at a single performance. The shows were done on a huge stage that was often overcrowded even though it could hold more than 200 people.

The expectancy of the crowd reached the point where I could walk on stage and within seconds have 50 to 100 people collapse in seconds and fall to the floor. All I had to do was go to the center of the stage, look over the entire crowd, raise my right hand and simultaneously drop it, and in a commanding voice shout "Sleep." This was a quick way to get the show moving, and that was important for full entertainment impact. The audience couldn't get enough of the show and enjoyed the humor of the volunteers' antics much more than how the actual hypnosis worked.

I was booked at the PNE by my new friend Mario Caravetta. He assured me I would return the following year, in 1981, to encore those incredibly successful performances. The PNE then went under a change of management, Mario left, entertainment buying policies changed, and my rebooking never materialized. This happened despite the fact that on a local radio phone-in show many people called in to say that the best attraction at the PNE had been "Romane."

Show Biz

During the late seventies and early eighties, I sported many outlandish outfits including sequins, brocade, silks, satins, bright flashy colors, fluorescent jackets that shone with blacklight, jackets with tiny mirrors that sent flecks like a mirror ball throughout the room. I even wore shoes with sparkly red toes as part of my extensive wardrobe. This was the style for an audience that was dazzled by the glitter and the extravagance one seldom sees in everyday life. Jewelry was also an important part of my costume, and I often received comments on my watch, which had twelve diamonds instead of numbers. I found it humorous that the watch got all the attention and only cost a few hundred dollars, while on my fingers were diamond rings that went virtually unnoticed yet their value was in the thousands.

I even went so far as to travel to Florida to see a popular designer named Michael. He had created outfits for Cher, Jimi Hendrix, and Sly Stone. I purchased one costume that was fitted with more than 2,000 rhinestones. The public enjoyed my fancy clothes, and I have to admit I enjoyed wearing them. Newspapers frequently commented on the glitter. Styles change though and the look is now more casual and contemporary—not everyone can dress like Elton John and get away with it.

Private Practice

In the late 70s, I opened a full-time office in a medical/dental office in Polo Park in Winnipeg. My clients came to me for private hypnosis sessions to help them lose weight; stop smoking; curtail foul language; develop confidence; improve memory, concentration, and coordination for sports; enjoy a more restful sleep; and even to enjoy housework.

One time I was seeing a well known Winnipeg boxer for hypnotherapy in order to improve his boxing skills. His sister decided to come for a session of hypnosis to motivate her to do housework. The hypnosis worked so well that she referred a friend. When I had had my fill of "enjoy housework" sessions, I made a recording called *Enjoy Housework*. This cassette has been popular and selling for more than 15 years.

One of the most interesting challenges that I encountered in private practice was the problem of an older gentleman who wanted to stop smoking. He was nearly deaf. I focused his attention upon my voice by turning off the lights and actually shouting directly into his ear for 45 minutes. At the end of the session, he said he felt fantastic. He became a permanent ex-smoker. But what was even more fascinating was that he said his hearing had never been better. Luckily, it was the last session of the day because my voice was simply no more.

It's All in the Voice

The quality of the voice is critical for efficient use of words not only in hypnotizing, but also in the following of suggestions. A reporter in Winnipeg once wrote a feature article about my presentation and labeled me as "The Man With The Velvet Voice." The voice must be sincere, caring, enthusiastic, uplifting, soft, permissive, or authoritarian as the application or individual may require. When I give suggestions to someone, simultaneously I vividly imagine them to be following the suggestions already. This does wonders for the voice inflections as well as the hypnotist's body language.

In the 1970s, 85 percent of my clients were interested in either losing weight or quitting smoking. In Manitoba, the winter months can be quite severe and I would have an increase in phone calls from smokers who were having difficulty breathing. It was hard for them to breathe such cold air into unhealthy lungs. I stressed self-hypnosis then as I do now. It is important for the client to acquire the ability to take control of his or her life without outside help. With self-hypnosis, the client feels that he controls his own destiny.

The most lasting impression I acquired by conducting private sessions was the realization that most of my clients didn't like themselves very much. This feeling was transmitted to me by the most attractive women; the most handsome men; the most financially successful, well-groomed and well-dressed clients who entered my office. The lack of self-confidence had no preference—social or economic. Many seemed to have the world in the palm of their hand but were empty inside. I found the most important therapeutic steps to be taken were to help these people appreciate themselves, life, and the world around them.

Clients have come to me from all over the world hoping that I will help them with hypnosis to stop smoking, lose weight, relieve anxiety, and overcome pain. Miracles do not always happen, but they happen often enough to make hypnosis worthwhile.

7

Living the Vision

My Vision

I remember reading somewhere that the essence of leadership is
to have a vision. I didn't decide to create a marketable vision out
of the blue, nor did it come to me in a dream. Rather, it simply
evolved over the years. Today it is more evident than ever that my
vision is to educate people to use the power of their minds to reach
their full potential and make their dreams come true.

Our brilliant unconscious mind with its warehouse of information and memories often reveals our inner self to us in our dreams.
Our unconscious is highly creative in our dreams because during
dreaming we have access to the accumulated memories of our entire
lifetime. The following came from my unconscious a few years ago,
in a dream:

"*A Hand In Love*"

I reached out my large warm hand.

You stood in my palm in mid-air.

You felt your own strength

and graciously stepped off my hand.

You did not need me anymore.

You had a healthier and more fulfilling life to live.

The work was done with love.

After I wrote the above, I had another dream about tricking the
grim reaper. I subsequently found a copy of "The Grim Reaper"
exactly as it was revealed to me in a dream or perhaps I should say
nightmare. In seconds my mind and body changed from a state of

82

powerlessness and perspiration to a feeling of tremendous strength
and success:

"The Grim Reaper"
You looked away from Death's eyes and
felt yourself growing weak and fading.
You looked Death straight in the eyes
and felt yourself coming back alive.
You looked Death squarely in the eyes
and you felt free.

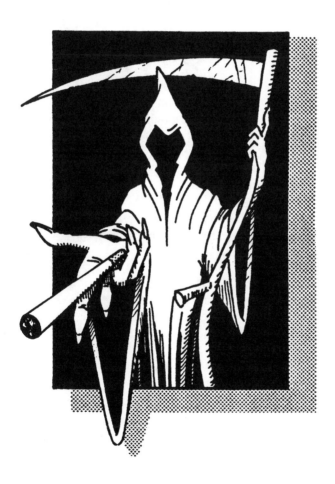

How to Remember Your Own Dreams

Before you fall asleep, affirm to yourself, "I will remember my dreams when I awaken." Keep a notepad next to your bed so that whenever you wake up you can write down the details of your dreams. Write down your feelings as well. This will help you to recall the location, characters, and other details. Before sleep, you can suggest to yourself that when you return to this dream world, you will be the writer and producer and you can easily change the events and outcome of the dream. Perhaps you will want to keep a journal of your dreams to notice themes or patterns. When you are asleep, but at the same time you are aware that you are dreaming, this is called lucid dreaming. With practice, you really can enter your dreams and change them to whatever you like.

Dream Exercise

Write on a paper specifically what you wish to dream about. Use plenty of details. Place the paper under your pillow and sleep on it. Talk to your self with your inner thoughts and believe you will have a dream related to your problem or goal. It may take one night or a few nights to see results. Trust your unconscious to do this for you.

Living the Vision

One of the reasons I feel so strongly about teaching people brain power methods is because of the powerful effect it's had on my own life. The more I learn, the more I want to teach and share with others.

Improving Your Health

At the age of five, while playing with three childhood chums in a railroad yard, I fell off the ladder of a train caboose. As I fell, my right leg bent behind my left leg and snapped like a match. I remember one of the boys, Ted, giving me some yellow and orange triangle shaped candies to distract me from my pain and shock. My young friends found an old worn out stretcher and carried me home on it. I screamed in pain all the way to my house. The adults who saw us assumed we were playing doctor and did not offer assistance. After my ride in the ambulance, I spent 49 agonizing days in traction in the hospital. Someone had taken my picture while I was hospitalized and that photo found its way to the front page of the Winnipeg Free Press. (It's amazing what was big news in the early 1950s!)

While my leg healed, it actually grew faster than my uninjured leg. When I reached my teens, my doctor decided to implant large U-shaped metal staples in my longer right leg to stop it from growing until my left leg caught up. The staples were stuck in my right knee bone. Due to the imperfections of this procedure, it wasn't unusual for these grotesque staples to pop out a fraction of an inch occasionally. Consequently, I continued to have more knee operations to restaple the knee bone and it was during one of the operations that I used my brain-power methods. I gave myself direct suggestions for rapid recovery, overall healing, and a healthy appetite. The hospital staff couldn't believe how quickly I recovered. I believe the key factor to my rapid recovery was programming myself with extremely powerful positive suggestions seconds before surrendering to unconsciousness from the anesthetic.

This is important. Just before loss of consciousness, the mind is fixated on the needle or gas while the doors to the subconscious are at the same time opening due to effect of the anesthetic.

Overcoming Pain

My subconscious has aided me many times when I experienced pain or discomfort. One night, for instance, I received a blow on the head, which resulted in a half-inch gash above my eyebrow. Without hesitation, I pinched the skin and imagined that I was in the desert with my skin drying and my blood clotting. I bandaged the cut, which could have used a stitch or two, and the skin sealed quickly thereafter.

Another night, I woke up with a splitting headache. I said to myself, "This headache is unnecessary. I'm going to get rid of it."

I asked my inner self: "Subconscious tell me what I have to do to get rid of my headache."

My subconscious said to me: "Chisel the pain out." I imagined I had a hammer and chisel and, in my imagination, I began to chisel the pain out of my head. After 20 seconds of chiseling, I was left with about 2 percent of the pain I experienced before, so I asked my subconscious again what to do. This time it said: "Blow it out." So I imagined a stick of dynamite and blew the remaining pain out. If this sounds weird, it did to me too, but it worked and fast!

It also is possible for one to disassociate oneself from pain by asking the subconscious to separate the painful area from the body.

This method can be used for burns, cuts, headaches, even after operations. A strong powerful self-suggestion can make it seem as if the painful area has been removed from the body or that it belongs to a stranger "over there." There is always a part of me that knows it isn't true, but I am able to convince myself so that 99 percent of my mind is convinced it is true.

This is done by focusing your concentration on the absorbing thought that you wish to implant. You may further intensify the self-suggestion by using as many other senses as possible. The more abundant that your sensory imagery is, the more powerful the self-suggestion should be as a rule. When I apply the technique, I first decide what I want to visualize then what I want to hear. I may add feelings, smells, and tastes as well.

I was able to see my leg after the operation, but I imagined that it was far away from me. It became someone else's leg, not mine, therefore someone else's pain. The pain either diminished or went away. Responses vary from time to time. I may imagine the leg is made of wood or leather and, therefore, it has no feeling. I may imagine that an anesthetic has been injected into the leg, and that it is numb. I may recall numbness from the feeling of cold ice locked into my memory and then transfer that memory feeling to my leg.

At other times, to block pain, I remember in vivid detail the freezing winters in Winnipeg. I transfer this memory of freezing to the painful area. The numbness of a dentist's injection of Novocain is also a good memory from which to draw relief. For a beginner to try these techniques, it might be helpful to submerse your hand in ice-cold water first. This sense memory of freezing cold can thereby be quickly established and thus available for future reference. At other times, I recall the coldness and numbness of rolling snowballs with bare hands.

Sometimes I try to make the best of pain by inventing a game. I tell the painful feeling to enlarge, to grow several times its actual area. For example, I might imagine that my ankle pain now extends to my foot, my leg, both legs, my mid-section, my upper body, the room, the house, the city, the province, the country, the continent, the world, and to infinity in outer space. I intensify the pain.

After this self-imagery, I reverse the above mental images and finally shrink the pain, bringing it to a pinpoint on the ankle until it finally disappears. It is often easier for the mind to first imagine pain, problems, and worries becoming worse before it can imagine them becoming better. This is why it is preferable to enlarge the problem and then shrink it down to make it less significant. It is much easier to gain control of pain by making it more intense, and then less intense.

Another technique is to focus upon the warmth of the pain. Or perhaps you may notice it as an interesting sensation. Ask your subconscious to allow the discomfort to leave you gradually in its own time. There is no need to give your inner mind a definite time limit. A good suggestion might be: "That feeling is leaving me now. It is beginning to fade, growing weaker, more dull, more boring. It may be completely gone or almost completely gone in one minute, 10 minutes, an hour, or a day. I do not know exactly when you will release it, my brilliant subconscious, but I do know that you will release it in your own time and way. Thank you for your great and wise help."

Solving Skin Problems

My relatives on my father's side, including my father and brother, have always had bothersome skin conditions such as eczema or rough skin on their fingers, hands, or arms. I began to get the same lesions on my fingers and arms through heredity, possible stress reactions, allergies, or some other unknown cause. When my skin condition did not clear, I tried an experiment. I looked at my clear hand that had no skin problem and asked my subconscious to make the hand with eczema look like the hand without eczema. The eczema skin condition disappeared within two days, and both hands looked the same. The eczema has never returned.

Hypnosis and Surgery

There is ample research available to document the fact that the unconscious mind records information even during the unconscious state of anesthesia during surgery. For example, a physician once remarked while making an incision on a female patient, "We sure have a lot of flab to cut through here." The patient had respected the physician for many years, but after awakening from surgery, she felt a deep resentment toward her physician. Only after having hypnotized the patient did the doctor come to the conclusion that she had been badly hurt by his insensitive remark. In hypnosis, but not in the waking state, the patient was able to recall the offending remark that the doctor made during surgery.

In another instance a physician, while speaking to a colleague during an operation said, "He will never walk again." After regaining consciousness, the patient could not walk. The physicians, however, had been referring to a different patient. The mind is so intensified during accidents, surgery, high fever, shock, during the announcement of the death of a loved one, and other traumatic events that the unconscious uncritically absorbs whatever is being said. In some hospitals there are signs over the operating room doors that read: "Be careful what you say, the patient is listening."

It distresses me when I hear someone say in the hallway of a hospital, "He doesn't look good" or "I don't think he'll make it through the night." When patients are entering surgery, they should be convinced of the competence of their physician and total support of their loved ones. While patients are hypnotized, it should be suggested that they have confidence in their doctor as well as that they will experience a rapid recovery. Positive chemicals are released within the body when we think positive thoughts, and if we plant positive suggestions that all these good things will happen following surgery, the patient is more likely to believe it. Positive direct and indirect suggestions given in and out of hypnosis may bring magical and startling results. I have seen it time and time again for decades.

I have a dear uncle named Neno who some years ago returned from a vacation with a deadly, unidentifiable blood disorder. This was not AIDS and long before the AIDS scare began. I wrote out positive suggestions on a card and gave them to his wife Dolly, who regularly read them to him. When I went to visit Neno, I gave him suggestions directly and indirectly. One of his physicians apparently had told him, "This disease is killing you." So when the priest, who came to administer the Last Rites, said "Are you ready, my son?" Neno whispered quietly (in a weak condition and dazed state), "I am." There seemed no question that death was nearby. His skin was black and blue from blood transfusions, his eyes blood-shot. He had lost a lot of weight and was weak. My loving aunt Minnie would not accept the priest's "good-bye ritual" and shouted "No! He's not ready!" In his groggy mental state, Neno feebly echoed her words replying, "No, I'm not ready." He was ready to say and do whatever he was told. That's hypnosis in its strongest form!

Neno's unconscious mind was in a hypnotic state that allowed him to be directed back and forth between life and death. Had my aunt Minnie not been there, Neno could well have accepted death. Dolly and Minnie gave their all in providing total love and care during Neno's lengthy illness.

Today I don't mind a little pain, for it can be a worthwhile experience. Why? On occasion, I have reframed pain into a positive experience by telling myself, "This is a good opportunity or challenge to practice my brain power techniques." Anger, self-pity, and complaining about the pain creates tension, and tension creates more pain. Relaxation and peace of mind reduce pain. When others show anger, you might say: "I love you."

If pain must occur, it is best to deal with it in a positive manner. I enjoyed trying to control pain in my youth. The day may come when I am even more thankful that I learned these techniques. When I was young, I had to have two good teeth extracted. I had protruding front teeth and space was required to move the teeth inwards with braces. I received an injection in my arm that was supposed to render me unconscious for the oral surgery. I decided, as an experiment, I would suggest to myself that nothing had been put into my arm. I told myself: "It's a placebo." I felt absolutely no effect from the drug. I remained wide awake, which stupefied the nurses. A nurse injected additional anesthetic into my arm. I decided this was a good time to go under—so I "let go" and became unconscious.

I must admit this was a foolish experiment, but it dramatically demonstrated the power of the mind over elements foreign to the body. Unfortunately, during this brain power experiment, I forgot to give myself suggestions for well-being after the operation. I awoke feeling extremely nauseated, regretting that the experiment had ever taken place.

CAUTION: *Be sure to make your physician aware of any brain power techniques you are using prior to the operation. He may be able to assist you in positively wording suggestions as well. Remember, you are in a hypnotically suggestive mental state just before "going under" the anesthetic.*

In the September 29, 1994, issue of the *Globe and Mail* newspaper, an article tells how a Welsh psychologist named Lalage Sanders plays audiotapes of smoking cessation messages to patients who are under general anesthesia. She told the British Psychological Society that although the 122 patients could not recall the tapes, those who received the anti-smoking messages definitely were influenced.

Going to the Dentist

Many people have such a tremendous fear of the dentist that they wait until their teeth are in terrible shape before they go. I prefer hypnosis to unnatural pain killers, if it is feasible, and usually do not take chemical freezing. Instead, I use brain power methods to overcome the pain. On several occasions, this meant sitting back and telling myself I was on a Waikiki Beach in Hawaii. In my imagination, the sound of the dentist's drill became the sound of airplanes bringing more tourists. The dental tools were straws from cool refreshing drinks that I sipped to quench my thirst.

While in the trance, I would tell my right hand it was numb and without any feeling or sensation. Then I would give myself suggestions of having a sensation of lightness in my right arm and hand. Then the right arm and hand would slowly float upwards with the hand brushing the side of my cheek and lips. Simultaneously, I would tell myself that I was transferring the numbness to my face and jaw.

When my dentist would tell me he was finished, I was almost disappointed that I couldn't stay on the beach a little while longer. I once had a tooth extracted with brain power methods as the sole anesthetic. My self-hypnosis was so effective that I was not even aware when the tooth was pulled out.

A good friend, John Parsons of Winnipeg, once told me that he never has taken anesthetic while at the dentist. When asked if he used self-hypnosis, he said, "No, I just will it." I suppose this may be a form of unconscious self-hypnosis. In my many years of studying hypnosis, I still believe perhaps the greatest form of self-control and change is through sincere prayer. When fully engaged in spiritual prayer, this is similar to a focused mental state of self-hypnosis. And I believe self-hypnosis is one of our many great gifts from the Creator.

Many aspects of religion involve the same principles of hypnosis. The most important are a belief in a higher power and the fixation of attention. To some extent when one speaks to one's subconscious as another being, it is a step to communicating with a higher power. (It is not necessarily the faith that is the higher power that inspires some, but the strength of the faith itself.)

Faith in oneself, for some, can be comparable to faith in a higher power. I visualize and conceive of the subconscious as a bridge of strength between our limited conscious mind and our brilliant universal consciousness, the Creator. The subconscious embodies the essence of our heredity, genetic knowledge, learned information, emotions, memories, impulses, potentials, self-healing, and mental, physical, and spiritual energy. One normally only reaches contact with one's subconscious brain power when one acknowledges and believes with their heart and mind that it is possible. Subconscious brain power is the gift of the Creator.

Fighting Fatigue

While on tour, I often did up to 29 presentations in a month. To battle fatigue, I developed a method to regenerate my energy. At the start of the tour, I would visualize myself feeling fantastic on the final day, whenever that would be. Specifically, I would visualize myself ending the tour after the last show or seminar feeling fantastic. Secondly, I would imagine myself at the end of the last presentation thinking about how I felt just great on every single day of the tour. This way my subconscious was able to take over my potential feelings of physical and mental vitality. If I neglected to practice this technique, I would instantly notice my energy draining. Tours can be grueling with up to 10 weeks being spent entirely on the road. This included dangerous roads on narrow cliffs, busy airports, blizzards, 40 below weather, and being away from loved ones.

The key to maintaining energy levels is to visualize vitality still strong on the last day of the tour and to be unconcerned with daily energy and strength. Just imagining enjoying life and feeling full of energy on the last day was all I needed to do. In addition, I could use my imagination to leap into the future while imaging that as I looked back into the past, everything had gone very well for me. This may set up a chain of events in your life that brings you the good luck and success that you earnestly desire. Likewise, negative imagery can bring you the reverse. Again, be careful what you focus upon, for you probably will get it. Just trust your subconscious mind to look after all the days before the last day of work or the day of realizing your desired goal.

Overcoming Insomnia

When I was touring, I was sometimes too wound-up after a show to sleep. Because of time zone changes and a demanding schedule, sleep was vital to my health and to my state of mind. To help me to fall asleep, I created mental imagery that would make me feel sleepy. Reading, for instance, always makes me tired. So, I sometimes imagined I was reading page after page, book after book. By time distortion, in seconds, it seemed as though I had been reading for 10 or 12 hours. Or, I imagined I was lying under a palm tree on a beach in Hawaii. If my body still felt tense, I imagined walking up a steep hill until I was too tired to walk another step. Sometimes, when I was too mentally exhausted to create my own images, I played one of my own relaxation tapes or sleep tapes and fell asleep while listening to the tape.

Here's another visualization I used to overcome insomnia. I imagine myself walking up a long steep hill and feeling more and more tired. At the top of the hill is an old Bavarian Hotel. I arrive after everyone is asleep, and the key is waiting on the desk for me. Feeling more and more tired, I go to my room. On the balcony of the room is a pile of rocks. I imagine myself throwing the rocks into the water below, one at a time. I watch the rings in the water become bigger and bigger, then smaller and smaller. I tell myself that as I watch the rings becoming larger and larger and then smaller and smaller that I feel more and more sleepy. Because I did this exercise so many times, I feel sleepy just thinking about it right now. I believe I may have learned this technique from Dr. William J. Bryan, Jr.

I am fortunate to have three healthy children, ages 12, 13, and 15, the youngest child being a son. When they were younger, occasionally they would have trouble falling asleep. I would lay down with the child and breathe in exact unison with him or her. My children usually fell asleep quickly and peacefully when this was done. Breathing is a powerful technique used in hypnosis. It is primitive and no language is necessary. Clinical psychologists and psychiatrists sometimes match breathing with their patient to create synchrony with the patient. Sometimes salespeople will match breathing, body movements, voice pace and tone, and other patterns to create a feeling of closeness with the client.

A Note about Sales Impulsion

As a young boy, I learned a technique for selling that often has proved effective. I present the information to the buyer and then just be quiet. However, while I am quiet, I mentally think the following thoughts over and over: "It's a great deal. I want it. That's fantastic. I want to take it home with me." Such thinking does wonders for your eyes, posture, and body language. In this way, you may influence the buyer at the most powerful level, the unconscious level. You can use this technique to sell items from pens to houses to ideas. Good luck applying this valuable technique.

More Insomnia Fighting Techniques

Another method that I found useful with insomnia clients was to teach them self-hypnosis and relaxation of the body with self-talk. When I had trouble sleeping as a teenager, I would remember the times that I was administered an anesthetic in an operating room. I would imagine I was back in the operating room, that I had received an anesthetic from a nurse and that I was mentally counting backwards from 100. Surprisingly, I found that I rarely went past the 90s before I fell asleep.

Sometimes my clients' minds are too active to sleep at night. I ask them to take out every dish in their cupboards and wash it. Being an onerous chore, this usually acts as a kind of aversive punishment. The client then finds he is sleeping better, because his inner mind says: "I'm not going to stay up or wake up early because I'll have to wash all those dishes again." This same method can be used for a multitude of unwanted behaviors. For confirmed insomniacs, sometimes it is best to accept the condition and use the time in a useful manner.

Many clients have told me that their marriage was under stress because one of the partners snored like a locomotive. My own father could sleep in a motel room next to me and his snoring was so loud that the sound came through the wall disturbing my sleep in the adjoining room. Many years ago, an assistant was touring with me and his snoring was so loud, that it was impossible for me to sleep. He insisted that he did not snore, so I recorded his snoring.

Then, for a lark, while he was sleeping, I played the tape recording back to him. He awoke angry and warned me in no uncertain terms that I should never do that again. Since he was much bigger than me, I suggested that he use a snore ball. Quite simply, this refers to sewing a small ball like a tennis ball on the back of the pajama top. Almost everyone snores while sleeping on their back. The snore ball is so uncomfortable that it keeps the sleeper off his back.

Myths Surrounding Hypnosis

The field of hypnosis is surrounded by misconceptions about its use. Hypnosis is centuries old and is now a valuable tool used by many physicians, psychologists, family therapists, psychiatrists, clergy, and dentists in their daily practice.

Hypnosis is not a religion or philosophy, nor is it witchcraft, occult, meditation, mind control, or superstition. The individual is not asleep or unconscious; he is alert and in control of the situation. There is nothing dark or mysterious about hypnosis. Hypnotized people are not zombies.

In the 1950s and early 1960s, even medical hypnotists were shunned by the medical profession. Claims were made that hypnosis had temporary effects and that it could damage one's mind. Hypnosis is now widely recognized as a valuable tool for healing and finding success in all areas of life. The number of people practicing hypnotherapy is escalating at an incredible rate. I've always said that a fad comes and goes. Hypnosis stays because it works. I believe that whatever you do, you'll do better with hypnosis.

Hypnosis is simply an altered state of consciousness, often characterized by relaxation and focusing of attention. When you are in that state of mind, you can act upon suggestions more readily than when you are fully awake.

We all go into self-induced hypnotic trances many times a day. For example, when you daydream and see yourself having fun on the beach, that's a form of transient hypnosis. Or sometimes you drive along your regular route to work and suddenly you wonder how you got there. Your mind has entered a *natural* hypnotic trance!

8

Questions and Answers

Is self-hypnosis dangerous?
No. In my experience, research, and studies in the field of hypnosis, I have not come across a single case in which a person experienced undesirable side effects due to the practice of educated formal self-hypnosis. As with every skill, formal training in the techniques of brain power methods is best.

CAUTION: *However great my faith is in the genius of our own unconscious mind, we must always allow the help of a physician to be close at hand. For example, if you have a mole and wonder if it is malignant, you should see a physician. Similarly, if you have recurring headaches, this could be a sign of a serious medical problem, so you should see your physician. By all means, enjoy the revelations of your own finely tuned unconscious, but remember to use traditional treatment as well.*

On the other hand, hetero-hypnosis (hypnotizing others) has resulted in a few problems when conducted by an amateur or inexperienced hypnotist. One should never hypnotize anyone without professional training, or after having studied hypnosis and psychology. Similarly, you should allow only a qualified professional hypnotist to hypnotize you.

Can anyone be hypnotized?
Yes. Any "normal" person can be hypnotized. Hypnosis is similar to the normal condition of daydreaming that everyone experiences. The key to successful hypnosis is *willingness* to be hypnotized. Almost anyone can learn or acquire the *skill* to be hypnotized by another individual.

Many years ago, stage hypnotists challenged that they could hypnotize *anyone*. One method of insuring success was to use chloroform. This is detailed in Ormond McGill's *Encyclopedia of Stage Hypnotism*. The hypnotist places a small bottle of chloroform in his right back pocket. The bottle has a two hole rubber stopper with two short glass tubes protruding. Rubber tubing is then attached to the glass tubes. One rubber tube runs up the hypnotist's right arm ending with another small glass tube. The other rubber tube coming out of the chloroform bottle goes to the hypnotist's left rear pocket and ends with a rubber squeeze bulb. The hypnotist then holds his right hand *near* the nose of the person to be hypnotized and suggests that he *imagine* breathing in chloroform. The *real* chloroform would make the client drowsy and more susceptible to hypnosis. Believing hypnosis was working then made it work even better.

Occasionally, a hypnotist will use aids such as guaranteed methods of proving to a client that he or she is suggestible. However, these are often illusions or muscle reactions that may occur even without any hypnosis. If used, the normal purpose is merely to give the client confidence and the belief that it is easy for him to be hypnotized. When you believe, then it is true for you.

Is hypnosis sleep?

No. Hypnosis is a condition of deep relaxation which is somewhere between being wide awake and asleep. Some subjects may drift off into ordinary sleep as the direct result of feeling deeply relaxed, but they then wake up shortly thereafter feeling terrific.

What if I don't come out?

Well, if someone did stay in hypnosis forever, I would be famous and they would be famous. It would be a first. No, everyone comes out of hypnosis.

Do I have to believe *hypnosis will work before it will help?*

On the contrary, I have hypnotized thousands of people, and many of those people were sceptical that they could be hypnotized by anyone. Many people have written and told me of their success in spite of the fact that they were leery of hypnosis or that they believed it would not be effective with them. Believing in hypnosis is definitely not always necessary to enjoy the benefits.

Do I have to really want to lose weight or quit smoking to make it work?

No, not at all. One of the foremost goals of effective self-help seminars is to motivate and excite the participant about the certainty of becoming a healthier person and reaching his or her goals. When I was doing a seminar in Vancouver, British Columbia, a lady told me she and half of her fellow workers were there only because their friends were. They had no real interest in quitting smoking, yet they were all successful in doing so. Hypnosis is an ideal method of communicating directly with the subconscious.

Once hypnotized, true reasons for the cause of a problem may be discovered. The real motivations may then be neutralized or side-tracked so they become satisfied in alternative healthy ways.

We also can teach the client self-hypnosis, which will help those who want to continue to achieve personal improvement independently of the hypnotist. Self-hypnosis helps sustain the feeling of relaxation, well-being, and confidence, which can result from planned positive suggestion.

Do people react differently to hypnosis?

Yes, they definitely do. There are various depths or levels of trance and some people are more suggestible than others. Without reinforcement, a post-hypnotic suggestion may or may not last. We can teach anyone self-hypnosis for any problem they seek to alleviate, and they are able to reinforce the suggestions themselves. Eventually, it becomes a permanent "re-conditioning" without need for further reinforcement.

I once read a study (source unknown) which stated that one exposure to an idea resulted in only 2 percent retention after 16 days. However, apparently 6 exposures over 6 days resulted in 62 percent retention for 15 years of life.

Why is it important to learn self-hypnosis?

For most people, just being hypnotized on a one-time basis is not the best solution to the problem. It is equally important that you learn how to apply the technique to your life for: (1) a greater feeling of personal achievement because you are accomplishing the improvement; (2) a greater feeling of *independence* because you will not have to visit a hypnotist repeatedly over a long period of time; (3) you may continue self-hypnosis for different problems throughout your life anywhere, anytime; (4) results are more likely to be more permanent; (5) self-hypnosis is more practical for you in terms of *both* financial and time considerations.

What is hypnosis like?

You are *not* asleep or unconscious. Your body becomes relaxed and your mind becomes super-aware and super-concentrated upon suggestions to help you. You may feel heavy, light, tingly, numb, or as though you're drifting or floating. For most, time seems to pass quickly. An hour might feel like 5 or 10 minutes. Hypnosis is a pleasurable rest and relaxation experience. Sensations vary from person to person. Sensations also vary greatly from session to session with the same person.

The real key to understanding hypnosis is that it is a mental state characterized by focused attention. When I was motoring to Palm Springs, I was quickly hypnotized by a policeman. I decided to take the long scenic route from San Diego. Coming down a country road to a stop sign, I wondered if I should turn right or left. I looked in my rear view mirror and thought, "What good fortune, a police car. I can ask directions." As I stepped out of the car, I noticed two police officers. The one in the driver's seat rapidly stretched both his arms out toward me. It was not a greeting. He was pointing his gun straight at me.

That gun somehow *focused* my attention and it looked larger than the ones I had seen in stores and museums. I raised my hands in the air, bent at the elbows. He shouted "What do you want?"

I smiled and said, "I'm a tourist."

He shouted, "You're committing a felony."

I said "Sorry," waved, and drove away. He did not seem too sociable, so I decided to turn left and get directions 10 miles further down the road. Fortunately, I was going the right way. I later learned that a few days earlier, a murder had occurred, which was still unsolved. The officers were perhaps a little nervous, as well as cautious.

I don't know why I wasn't frightened, even though that was the first time a gun had ever been pointed at me. However, when I first saw the gun, I was in hypnosis for a couple of seconds because my mind was focused.

People go into hypnosis spontaneously every day. Let me give you some examples of everyday hypnosis with focused attention:

- Driving your car along the road while your mind is focused upon a problem and you drive past the exit you intended to take.
- Becoming so lost in a book, a movie, a concert, or music that you temporarily forget about everything around you.
- Blocking out everything around you while writing a story or a letter. When you're taking an examination, doesn't time seem to drift away rapidly?
- Forgetting where you parked your car; where you placed your keys or glasses only two minutes ago; forgetting every word on a page of a book you just read; lighting a second cigarette and forgetting you already have one lit and sitting in the ashtray. These are examples of deeper levels of hypnosis characterized by amnesia or forgetting.
- Looking for something, but not seeing it, even though it is "staring you in the face."
- Driving for miles without noticing the scenery and wondering where the time went.
- Staring blankly with glassy eyes and motionless body lost in thought.
- Searching for something already in your hand.

Sometimes I tell people: "I am not going to hypnotize you to do anything. Instead, I am going to *dehypnotize* you from the beliefs and negative self-suggestions that are causing your problems."

Hypnotic trances and altered states of consciousness can be induced easily by a flashing strobe light (not to be used with individuals with epilepsy); music, especially certain African, Indonesian, Indian, and West Indian music; repetitive drumming sounds; dancing; deep breathing; isolation tanks; mediation; massage; spas and hot springs; even a ride in Disneyland through darkness with a sudden drop can cause an altered state of consciousness and a "hypnotic flash." It is during that time of focused attention where hypnotic suggestions have their greatest impact.

How do hypnotists hypnotize in seconds?

A favorite method of mine is to:

1. Ask a client if he is ready to be cooperative or willing to be hypnotized.
2. Give prehypnotic conditioning suggestions: "I'm going to hypnotize you. Your body will relax completely; your eyes will close;

and your head will fall forward. Please push your right palm down on my left palm."

3. Once his attention is fixed, I quickly pull my hand away.
4. Right then, I fire the suggestion: "SLEEP!"
5. I continue rapid-fire relaxation suggestions, such as "Your body is heavy like rock. You remain in hypnosis. You hear every word I say. Follow every positive suggestion that I give to you. Forget about your body. Let your mind drift, dream, and float."

At the point of my hand being pulled away, his conscious mind is suddenly diverted. At that split second, and because he has willingly given his permission to be hypnotized, he goes into hypnosis. This can sometimes be abbreviated to a couple of seconds, such as "Look into my eyes (fixed gaze by both of us). Sleep!"

Does music enhance hypnotizing?

I have found over the years that music, as well as sound effects can have a tremendous impact in increasing concentration and suggestibility. The body is an electromagnetic organism. Sound is an electromagnetic vibration. Sound, specifically the right kind of music, can heal the body, mind, and spirit. Music can evoke calm breathing, a relaxed heartbeat, and alpha brain waves. By evoking the relaxation response with sound, less anesthetic is needed in surgery.

A parent turns the lights down low and rocks and sings her child to sleep. My uncle Neno brought me a wonderful gift of wind chimes from Mexico. I suspended them on my balcony and every time I hear the wind chimes tingling, I feel relaxed.

Music Relaxation Exercise

Play relaxing music, close your eyes, and completely relax. Point the soles of your feet toward the CD player's speaker. Just listen and let your mind focus only on the music. Let your mind drift, dream, and float.

Do you black out when you are hypnotized?

Not at all. Everyone who is hypnotized is *super-aware* of what is happening. To follow a hypnotist's suggestions, the hearing sense has to remain alert.

Will I do something against my moral standards?

No, you will not accept a suggestion that you do not wish to accept because of your *subconscious censor.* People can even lie when under hypnosis. Hypnosis instruction, as given at professional self-hypnosis training seminars, is totally safe and enjoyable.

Will I reveal all my personal business while I am under hypnosis?

Again, you won't reveal anything you don't wish to. No one spontaneously begins speaking of "skeletons in the closet." Hypnosis is not a truth serum. Because of greater imaginative abilities in hypnosis, people can tell lies far better when hypnotized than when out of a trance.

What's the difference between clinical and stage hypnosis?

Stage hypnosis is meant to entertain while the purpose of clinical hypnosis is to change thoughts, feelings, and behavior for a healthier life. To be entertaining, stage methods of hypnotising must be more rapid than clinical methods. Although clinical methods may be slower, they usually are far more successful in terms of the percentage of people successfully hypnotized. People not hypnotized on stage usually can be hypnotized easily by a good clinical hypnotherapist. To be entertaining, the stage hypnotist must have a rapid pace at his show. This limits the number of people who can be hypnotized. Many people require a slower more lengthy hypnotic induction as may be done in a clinical situation.

What is the difference between positive thinking and hypnosis?

Positive thinking deals with the conscious mind (thinking) while hypnosis deals with the subconscious mind (emotions). Emile Coué, the French psychotherapist, became famous for his positive self-affirmation: "Every day in every way, I am getting better and better." He taught in Europe and in the United States emphasizing how the imagination could effect self-healing and even organic changes.

An interesting story relates to Coué's visit to New York. Meeting an old friend there, Coué inquired, "How's everything, Pierre?"

Pierre said, "My uncle is very sick."

Coué replied, "No. No. No. Your uncle just *thinks* he is sick."

Two weeks later, when they met again, Coué asked: "How is your uncle?"

Pierre moaned, "He *thinks* he's dead."

Current research does suggest that a positive attitude by a patient will contribute to a faster recovery. In addition, if the healer such as his physician expects a rapid and full recovery, this vastly increases the chances of good health. In other words, believe and it may well be so! Think of your brain as a bowl. Decide to pick up a beaker or pitcher labeled "Positive Suggestions" and pour some of its contents into the "bowl" every day.

Hypnosis is more effective than positive thinking because it deals with a problem at its roots. Your subconscious mind is more powerful than your conscious mind. For example, perhaps your conscious mind wants to quit smoking but your subconscious doesn't have any concerns or desires about quitting. Thus, hypnosis allows positive ideas and suggestions to enter your inner subconscious mind. The subconscious part of the mind accepts, believes, and has faith in the suggestions and acts upon them without analyzing or questioning the suggestions. Of course, the subconscious has a censor, which blocks dangerous or immoral suggestions.

How do you help people lose weight or stop smoking?

One of the first things I do is to motivate them by live lectures and by indirect suggestions during the lecture itself. In the live lectures, I may discuss how powerful the hypnosis has been with past clients. I talk about the benefits of losing weight or stopping smoking. It is important that the client personally *wants* to lose weight or quit smoking, rather than to merely please her friends or loved ones. Of course, *loving* support from her friends is also of great help.

Misconceptions about hypnosis can create a fear of being hypnotized, and they generally must be eradicated before any hypnotizing will be successful. It also is important to create a certain positive atmosphere or mood to assist the client to achieve the right frame of mind. To do this, I teach clients to believe in themselves and to love their body so much that they want to protect and look after it. Mastering stress control also is extremely important. Valuable techniques may be learned to be calm and relaxed under almost any circumstances and to achieve a feeling of control over one's life.

In hypnotizing, believing in oneself is important to the client's state of normal conscious awareness. Then I feed positive visual images into the client's subconscious. For smokers, I may input visual images to encourage the client to visualize himself as a non-smoker. Images such as friends complimenting him on his success, seeing his lungs looking and feeling healthier, and feeling much more energy as a breather of clean, fresh air.

In hypnosis, the deep relaxation that you feel allows pain killer beta endorphin chemicals or "happy chemicals" to be released. The right hypnotic suggestions can relax the mind and body and make us more receptive to suggestion. Lastly, hypnosis helps break the unhealthy habit's connections—for example, connections between coffee and smoking, alcohol and smoking, stress and smoking, or boredom and smoking. These habit connections may be broken by positive suggestion, visual imagery, and metaphors directed to the unconscious mind.

Weight control, like smoking, is assisted by a lifestyle change as well as hypnosis therapy. A researcher once tested 3,000 weight loss methods and discovered that the *only* way to lose weight is to reduce calorie intake and to increase exercise. My hypnosis seminars teach clients healthier eating habits, stress control, and appreciation of his or her body which brings expectations of success, and most importantly, self-confidence.

Hypnosis is a gift to mankind to motivate the spark within us, to exalt and perpetuate the desire for change. However, if there is no spark, no initial motivation at all, it is more of a challenge to help someone. We can turn a spark into a fire, but it is difficult to make a fire without a spark. When one wants to change, hypnosis becomes a great lever to multiply the client's motivation and release inborn mental powers of hidden knowledge, creativity, and self-discipline.

I often combine numerous other techniques with hypnosis to boost the success rate of my sessions. This may include a variety of practical self-control methods, behavioral conditioning methods, and stress control techniques. However, hypnosis, creative visualization, auto-suggestion, and various other brain power techniques remain the most used techniques that create change in my clients. It is also important to understand that knowing what to do often does not ensure doing it. Every dusty exercise bike will validate that fact.

The problem begins in the mind and can only be solved in the mind. Today's professional hypnotist merely acts as a facilitator who creates a mental atmosphere for enhancing the client's motivation, imagination, expectancy, and the release of inborn strength for limitless possibilities of self-healing and self-enhancement.

Are there many female hypnotists?

When I began many years ago, there were few female hypno-tists, yet now there are thousands. Like many professions in the past, somehow most women did not see hypnosis as suitable to their femininity. But as women began entering careers that were tradition-ally "male," more and more female hypnotists sprung-up. Today there are thousands of females who enjoy practicing hypnosis. Their natural, warm, caring nature becomes a valuable healing asset.

Why is hypnosis a valuable tool?

Hypnosis can be used to relax, to relieve pain, to alleviate anxi-ety, and to recall certain events. It has been effectively used to relieve pain in terminal cancer, in minor and major surgery, and in childbirth. In dental work, hypnosis is helpful in controlling anxiety and pain, and it can help reduce the amount of analgesic drugs needed in such work. Excessive eating and smoking can be elimi-nated as well as most other unhealthy habits. Hypnosis also can be a helpful way to treat neuroses.

Simply being in hypnosis, without having been given any spe-cific hypnotic treatment suggestions, will result in a tranquilizing effect on the body. Just being placed in hypnosis for a few days for mental rest and rejuvenation in order to alleviate anxiety may be a tremendous overall healer for the mind, body, and spirit.

A study by Dr. Ichiro Kawachi, assistant professor of health and social behavior at the Harvard School of Public Health, links high anxiety and sudden cardiac death. Apparently, men who complain of high anxiety are up to *six* times more likely than calmer men to suffer sudden cardiac death. By comparison, the risk of sudden cardiac death among smokers was only twice as high as it was among nonsmokers.

Another great application for hypnosis is in the field of educa-tion. Most students can be helped with hypnotherapy to increase concentration, sharpen recall abilities, and improve study habits. Hypnosis also may help to alleviate examination anxiety. There are many such beneficial uses of hypnosis that are not medically related, such as building self-confidence, enhancing talents, and even in achieving maximum excellence in athletics.

Is hypnosis used by the medical community?

Yes. Hypnosis is a valuable tool in virtually all areas of medical treatment. Morning sickness, insomnia, chronic pain, and migraines can all be reduced through hypnosis. Hypnosis has been used in successfully treating constipation, bed wetting, and some skin conditions which are stress aggravated. It has been said that the skin mirrors the emotions.

Some hypnotists use hypnosis to help eliminate phobias such as fear of flying, fear of driving, fear of public speaking, fear of needles, or perhaps the fear of just tensing up at the sound of a dentist's drill. There are also some patients who have to forgo anesthesia for medical reasons. Hypnosis can be vital for such patients. Being unconventional for most, hypnosis is often the last method chosen, the last resort. Often it does work like a miracle!

Can hypnosis help you locate misplaced items?

Yes, I have induced trances in clients to facilitate the remembering of past events and to locate misplaced items. Many people give themselves the negative self-suggestion: "I'll hide this where no one can find it." What they should say is, "I'll hide this where *only I* can find it." As a result of such negative self-suggestion, people may lose valuable jewelry, money, and mementos. I have been approached by clients on numerous occasions to assist in locating such items. We often have been successful in tracking down lost articles. One method used to assist in finding something is to hypnotize the person and with the aid of regression, to retrace the route he took when hiding the object. We may develop a detailed scene of the person hiding the object, encouraging the client to use as many senses as possible. As an alternative, I might tell the hypnotized client to have a dream about the missing object and to wake up with a memory of that dream.

Another successful method to locate lost objects uses Chevreul's pendulum. This can be made with string tied to a ring or fish weight. I tell the client to hold the end of the string with the weight dangling directly in front of him or her. The client is told not to move his or her hand but to let the string or weight move in whatever direction it will. The client can be given a list of questions about the lost object and trained so that the moving pendulum answers the questions automatically. A code system may be set up with the subconscious mind.

For example, the hypnotized person may be told that if the

pendulum moves from side to side the answer is no. If the pendulum moves forward to backwards, then the answer is yes. The pendulum moving in a circle could indicate uncertainty, while a motionless weight could mean "I don't want to answer that question right now." This last option is added to allow the possibility of the subconscious mind answering the question at a later date, if an answer is not immediately available. This technique may be used in the lightest trance and even without a trance.

Do you have to be relaxed to be in a trance?

No, one doesn't necessarily have to be relaxed. All that is needed is a focused mind. People go into trances when in a state of terror, shock, high fever, and emotional stress; while watching TV; while lost in a good book; or while absorbed in beautiful music. However, relaxation is a good aid to hypnosis when tension is an obstacle in focusing the mind.

How much of my session will I remember?

While you are in a hypnotic state, you will remember most or all that went on during the session. Some people remember everything, while others remember only parts of their session. It's like awakening in the morning and not remembering everything you dreamed about during the night. Hetero-hypnotic trances experienced at deeper levels have often resulted in clients not remembering anything at all. Total amnesia normally occurs only during hetero-hypnosis due to the deeper levels attained. Sometimes, a hypnotherapist will ask the client to create an amnesia for therapeutic reasons. Some therapists believe that changes may be stronger if the person does not remember the positive hypnotic suggestions given. That is, if the suggestions are forgotten and locked inside the subconscious mind, then the conscious mind cannot defeat them since there is simply no conscious awareness of the suggestions.

Some people have amnesia after a *self-hypnotic* session. Perhaps they were so relaxed that they entered a normal sleep and, consequently, forgot most of the session. By suggesting to yourself that you will remember your thoughts and sensations after a session, you will. However, vivid memories of a session are not at all essential for suggestions to be effective. Many of my clients spontaneously forget a substantial part of the hypnotic session.

When you are hypnotized, you may hear a telephone ring, the

sound of birds, or the hum of an air-conditioner. These sounds need not disturb you. When you are hypnotized, it is often useful to imagine that any sound you hear (except an emergency, of course) is relaxing you deeper and deeper. If the telephone rings, you may answer it, talk briefly, and immediately return to your trance. On the other hand, you may suggest to yourself that with every ring of the telephone, you will go deeper into hypnosis.

What precautionary suggestions should be given to hypnotized people?

The following are recommended:

1. You can only be hypnotized when you wish to be hypnotized and only by a qualified practitioner.

2. You will never be hypnotized while operating a vehicle or heavy machinery or while in a situation where it may be dangerous for you.

3. No one may take advantage of you under hypnosis. You only follow suggestions which are for your greatest good, health, and happiness.

4. If any emergency were to occur while you are in hypnosis, you instantly would come out of hypnosis feeling clear-headed, alert, refreshed, and full of energy. Should you feel that you need any other suggestion to protect you while you are in the state of hypnosis, that suggestion is given to you now and takes full, complete, and thorough effect over your mind, body, and spirit.

5. It also is beneficial to suggest that you may return instantly to the hypnotic brain power state with a certain cue, such as a specific word, gesture, movement, or sound. For example: "When you rub your thumb and index finger together, you instantly will return into hypnosis." Another example: "When you (or I) count from 10 to 1, you instantly will be in hypnosis." This type of post-hypnotic suggestion may be applied both with hetero-hypnosis and with self-hypnosis to dramatically shorten the time needed to be rehypnotized.

How much time is required for brain power training sessions?

For the first few weeks, 20 to 30 minutes for each session is advised. After you are well practiced with the methods, you will be able to hypnotize yourself in a few minutes or even seconds. The best time to have a session is before you fall asleep, while in bed.

However, if you tend to fall asleep before completing your session, then do your sessions during the day, or while sitting up in a straight-back chair. Too much comfort may produce ordinary sleep. Obviously you cannot give yourself hypnotic suggestions if you fall asleep too soon.

If you have the time you can do two or three sessions a day. The number of sessions required to overcome a problem is related to the type of problem, its severity, the length of time it has existed, and other individual factors such as motivation.

How successful are brain power methods?

Hypnosis is not the answer to all problems nor is it beneficial in all applications. However, for breaking bad habits and general self-improvement, hypnosis can be extremely successful. With *professional* hypnosis, most people will notice improvement or total elimination of their problem. Often, only light hypnosis is required for noticeable success. Light hypnosis is easily attained by most people. I urge you to maintain your enthusiasm even if you do not succeed with hypnosis immediately. While practicing your exercises during your first few sessions, many competing thoughts may go through your mind such as: "Am I doing this right?" or "Am I hypnotized?" or "Is it working? I hope it's working. When will it work?" These thoughts may prevent you from entering a hypnotic trance and enjoying the benefits, unless you take command. Just allow these negative thoughts to withdraw from your mind and think only about relaxing and the beneficial suggestions you want your subconscious to accept.

Here's a method I sometimes use to calm my mind: Imagine a calm lake with beautiful blue water. Now imagine sticks floating in the water, drifting away never to be seen again. These vanishing sticks may represent your unwelcome thoughts, which are interfering with your mind focusing.

If I hypnotize you, your mind will not be blank at all times. Even if you are deeply hypnotized, your mind will sometimes wander. In such a case, just bring your attention back to the hypnotist's voice. If you eliminate worry about your mind wandering, it will wander less and less. Your mind is just busy tossing about the suggestions of relaxation and those specifically designed to help you to change your thoughts, feelings, and behavior.

The less that you care about your doubts about success, the more the doubts will want to leave you. Remember that most things you worry about never happen. And the things that will happen with absolute certainty will happen regardless of what you do, so they certainly are not worth worrying about.

After the first couple of sessions, the suggestions you have been implanting may be only lightly impressed upon your mind. Similar to advertisements that are repeatedly shown, suggestions become more effective after numerous repetitions or reinforcements. Even after your problem has been eliminated, your self-suggestions should be periodically reinforced for *permanent* results. It is most beneficial to "over-learn" in hypnosis.

What is your favorite method of hypnotizing others?

After more than 35 years of hypnotizing others, I have found the following formula to be the most successful with the most people. This is an almost fail-safe technique of induction, and it is rare when someone is not hypnotized by this method. In the case of a failure, this normally is due to the client having excessive psychological difficulties occurring in his life at that time. Here are the steps of my most powerful group hypnosis method:

1. Dispel all general misconceptions about hypnosis to eliminate potential mental blocks. For example, I might say:

"In hypnosis, you are not asleep. You will hear me all the time. If you do not hear me, please let me know. It means that you are deaf or dead. I cannot possibly help you if you do not hear me. So, you will hear me all the time.

"Everyone always comes out of hypnosis. I have hypnotized hundreds of thousands of people and I have yet to return to a city and see someone walking down the street with their arms outstretched. If you do not come out of hypnosis, we will both be famous, because that has never happened at anytime in the past.

"When you are being hypnotized, you should keep your eyes closed, as this will help you to focus your attention upon my voice. You will be *super* aware of my voice, not unaware. Your mind will not be a blank. You will hear everything that I say. Your mind may wander from time to time, but that is okay. It is possible for your mind to wander, even if you are in the deepest hypnosis. You may even forget parts of the experience, but that is okay. The positive suggestions will go right on helping you, beyond your awareness.

"You can move or change your position while you are in hypnosis. However, you may not feel like moving. You may forget certain parts of the experience; however, that is all right. The positive suggestions, although possibly forgotten by your conscious mind, will be remembered, followed, and acted upon by your inner subconscious mind.

"Here is the secret of going into hypnosis. Just let your body go floppy, loose, limp, limber, like a rag doll, like this. *There is no need to 'try hard'. Just let it happen.*" (At this point, with my own body, I often demonstrate how to let go in all the muscles.)

2. I ask the client to tense up every muscle of his body for a few seconds and then to relax all the muscles.

3. I ask the client to inhale three deep breaths, breathing in relaxation and breathing out tension.

4. I ask the client to moisten his lips with his tongue and to just let his mouth stay open a little, to just let the jaw hang loose. I then ask the client to relax the muscles around his eyes so much that they simply will not open. The client is now asked to test his eyes to make sure that they do not work. If the eyes open, the client is told to keep doubling the relaxation of the eyes until they no longer work. I might even ask him to yawn, as this helps to relax the throat muscles and, thus, quiet the speech and thinking part of the mind. Also, additional oxygen enters the body to aid in the relaxation.

5. I may ask the client to recall the most relaxing moment in his life, perhaps on a mountain top, in a warm bath, in a field, upon a beach, or someplace else chosen by the client. I then ask him to really be there with all his senses and his imagination.

6. Next, the client is told to allow the relaxation in the eyes to spread through the rest of the body, starting with the head and ending with the tips of the toes.

This is the essence of my formula that can be successful with almost anyone. Of course, one should have professional training before using this process, which has been abbreviated in format and is strictly for illustration.

How can I help myself to be hypnotized rapidly?

The best advice I can give to you is to simply let your body go floppy, loose, and relaxed. Do not care if you are hypnotized, for not caring about the outcome will eliminate the frequent, endless interference of asking yourself over and over: "Am I really hypnotized? Is it working? I hope I'm hypnotized! When will it work?" Having worked with hundreds of thousands of people, I have found that simply telling clients the above will assist virtually anyone to be hypnotized easily. Again, just treat hypnosis as a special time to simply relax and to focus your mind upon success. Then trust the subconscious to bring you the success which you desire.

Experiment in Letting Go to Be Hypnotized

Hold your right or left hand in a fist as tight as you possibly can. Keep squeezing tighter and tighter. Notice the whiteness in your hand. Do not let go until you are too physically tired to hold it tightly any longer. After you finally let go, notice how much better your hand feels while relaxed in contrast to when it was tense. Similarly, when you allow yourself to let go to enter the brain power state of mind, the process becomes most easy for you.

9

The Power of Positive Thinking

P sychologists have maintained that whatever we think the most about, we will become. Years ago, William James said that an idea held strongly and powerfully in the mind will tend to realize itself. In other words, whatever you pay attention to in your life, positive or negative, that energy field will grow stronger. Sales motivational coaches tell us that if we imagine ourselves as successful long enough and hard enough, we will become successful. Napoleon said, "Imagination rules the world."

If we surround ourselves with positive-thinking people, we are more likely to think positively. Think of the happy feelings and personal magnetism a good entertainer projects and generates to his audience. If you are confident of your abilities, other people will have confidence in you and give you a chance to prove yourself. If you present yourself with a lack of faith in your capabilities, you will not even be given a chance to show your talent.

Dealing with a Feeling of Failure

Successful people have one secret in common. Every time they fall, they get up and try again. I remember past events so that I may learn from them, but I avoid dwelling upon them. I will no longer allow myself to ever feel a failure at anything. However, I will allow myself to have setbacks or mistakes. Do your best to eliminate the word failure from your vocabulary. Setbacks in your past may teach you to be more compassionate with others who have similar problems. Your setbacks also may give you the gift of empathy, which enables you to help others to solve the problems you once had. Never feel guilty for anything you have done in the past, but rather use it as positive experience to assist you in the future. My belief is that one should make amends to the best of his ability and make a decision to do better in the future.

Too many people waste valuable energy ruminating about the pain of the past or worrying about the "what ifs" of the future. Pondering painful past experiences only releases mental pictures of past hurts, negative chemicals, and the reliving of past negative emotions. If you spend your valuable time thinking about how you are going to fail or about what is going to go wrong, you may be setting yourself up for sickness and failure. In other words, "that which I hath feared hath come upon me."

I had a relative who persisted in recalling a painful marriage and divorce for about 40 years. He died of a heart attack. Others will keep reminiscing about negative past experiences being unable to forgive and forget the event. A negative energy is then created to poison their new relationships. It may be hard to *completely* forget painful experiences with someone, but if one *allows* the transition to happen, it will. You may never completely forget, but if you do not forgive, you can forget the new relationship.

Focus upon the expectation of harmony, happiness, and success for your future. Focus on the present and what is now working for you. Forgiveness may bring inner peace. Negative experiences with someone can be replaced over time with new positive experiences.

Personal misfortune can leave you bitter, or it can leave you better. The words of Ella Wheeler Wilcox, the 19th-century American author, express it best: "The world is round, and the place that seems like the end may only be the beginning."

Sometimes the bad things in life turn out to be good in the end. As Alexander Graham Bell once said: "When one door closes, another door opens. But we so often look so long and so regretfully upon the closed door, that we do not see the ones which open for us."

Often a client will ask me to help him to overcome a habit or a recurring unpleasant memory. For example, trying hard not to smoke or trying hard not to overeat is like trying hard to forget the word elephant. One technique that I use might be to ask a client to imagine a hanging sign that says: SMOKING: THAT IS THE PAST.

A person with a strong faith in God may be told: "Rest the problem in the hands of God and just let it melt away. God will solve that problem for you in his or her own unique way. Remember, you cannot place your problem in God's hands, then take it back."

Replace Unhealthy Habits with Healthy Ones

It also is often helpful to replace an unhealthy habit with something positive, rather than just taking the habit away. Changes are more likely to be permanent with healthy substitutes replacing the unwanted behavior.

Throughout the 1970s, I did hundreds of entertainment shows in schools, colleges, fairs, exhibitions, and conventions throughout the U.S. and Canada. The popularity of the shows brought me theatrical and financial success. In 1981, a recession hit and budgets tightened. Ticket sales decreased rapidly, the demand for hypnotic shows was almost zero and few were willing to hire me. I remember my accountant telling me it was time I faced reality and changed career directions before I went bankrupt.

I knew I couldn't give up so easily. I sat down and wrote out all of my assets and interests. One that shone through was my knowledge and experience with helping people achieve self-improvement through hypnosis. I researched public interest, trying to find what the public demanded at this time. I discovered the two services that were extremely popular were stop smoking programs and weight loss clinics. I decided to develop a series of seminars to help people stop smoking and lose weight based on my interests, knowledge, and experience.

In fact, a new door did open that brought me even greater personal happiness. During the 1960s and early 1970s when I wanted to engage in serious hypnosis to help people, few folks were interested. This was one of the reasons why I decided to expand my career as a theatrical hypnotist. I also enjoyed making people laugh until tears streamed down their cheeks. It helped people to forget their daily worries and cares for awhile. Laughter results in happier and healthier people.

Audiences at the concerts loved to see their friends hypnotized. When the hypnotized people felt the surge of confidence to be able to do most anything, including comical stunts, these antics literally made spectators fall out of their chairs laughing. Some people said their sides hurt from so much laughing. These antics were talked about by audience members for weeks after the show.

114

Many years ago, at one of my entertainment concerts, a gentleman said to me: "You have this remarkable gift to make people do almost anything. Why don't you use it to help people instead of asking them to do all these comical things?" His comment echoed in my mind and that was one of the major events that made me change careers.

Now at last, I could pursue my love of serious hypnosis to help thousands of people. Although, I conducted a large number of hypnosis seminars in the 1970s, this was only a fraction of the number of seminars I conducted across Canada in the 1980s and 1990s.

I felt a greater sense of self-fulfillment by using my time to conduct these self-help seminars. More satisfied in a personal way, I was rewarded financially with a reasonably good income as well. It's amazing how many people continue to ask me: "Can you really make a living doing that?"

I still enjoy the theatrical shows, but I am glad I have the opportunity to continue to practice what has always been my first love: helping other people. The benefits of my seminars reach far beyond the people who attend them. For example, because I helped a person stop smoking, a child with asthma or a pet may find the air easier to breathe.

Trouble isn't always trouble. We may experience adversity and setbacks for a purpose, even if we don't know what the purpose is at the time. Our *reactions* to our circumstances and the choices we make are more important than what happens to us. We can choose to moan, "Oh I'm just a failure." Or, we can choose to examine our lives, look for a positive purpose in our circumstances and take specific steps that will set us on the path to a better and happier life. The choice is ours.

Someone once said to me, "If every door you knock on in a building shows no response, try a different building." For example, if you have an occupation which seems impossible to make a living with, perhaps it's time to stop banging your head against the wall and try a new occupation. Simply put, if what you are doing is not working, stop doing it and try something different.

Worry

Mark Twain once said, "I am an old man and have known many troubles—most of which never happened." Research tells us that

Mark Twain was right; most of the things people worry about never do happen. Excessive worrying is an unhealthy mental habit that you can change.

Remember, you became a worrier by practicing worry. You can become free of worry by practicing the opposite and stronger habit of faith. Every morning when you arise, say to yourself: "The Creator has given me another wonderful day to enjoy." Practice saying something positive concerning anything about which you have been creating negative self-talk. For example, never say, "This is going to be a terrible day." Instead affirm, "This is going to be a *wonderful* day." Never say, "I can't do that." Instead affirm, "I *will* do that, and *I will do it well.*"

The beginner will not be able to use these techniques with the magic and precision of a trained hypnotherapist. Like a musician, a hypnotherapist's skills are carefully sharpened through years of practice.

Spending time fretting over things takes time away from your life and could result in nervous problems such as excessive smoking, overeating, insomnia, and nail-biting. Or, if a person has an unhealthy habit such as smoking, the more he or she worries about it, the more serious the habit becomes. In fact, worrying about smoking can cause you to smoke even more. A vicious circle is established.

Pondering over one's life is fine, but continual reminiscing is only a waste of time. Perhaps it is best to think of your troubles as a problem and then work at solving them. If the problem can't be altered or solved, it should be calmly accepted and forgotten. Think of the present and the future for that is where you will be spending the rest of your life. Always retain hope for better days ahead. *It isn't productive to allow your mind to be preoccupied with your troubles.* Think of a way to alter them. If that doesn't work, forget them and get on with enjoying life!

If you had worries before you read this section, and if you feel better already, do not rest on your laurels. Read this section over and over until it is branded into your mind. Read it until you no longer just have the thoughts, but *the thoughts have you* and will never let go. More importantly, write on a piece of paper the words or phrases that have the strongest effect to make you feel better. You will know when you have the right words or phrases when they create an *emotional* feeling of well-being within you. After you have read these phrases several times, place yourself into the brain power state of mind, self-hypnosis. While you are in self-hypnosis, allow one of these powerful phrases and feelings to echo in your mind and flow through your body from the top of your head to the tips of your toes. Focusing steadily upon one clear, crisp, multi-sensory image or affirmation at a time will generate steadier concentration and greater success.

Would you like to help others cure their worry habits? *By helping others* to overcome worry, you can achieve a greater feeling of power over your own worry. As you help others, so you help yourself. Be positive when you are talking with others. This isn't to say be fake or unrealistic, but try to see the good in things. It's fruitless to harp on the negative things in life, so search for the love and the good in the world.

Excess tension often results in similar problems. When you worry, tension mounts. The increase in tension causes a more severe problem which in turn increases tension. The goal is to break the vicious circle via hypnotic suggestion. If an overweight person, for example, is trying to eat less but overeats at one particular meal, he may feel guilty, depressed, or angry with himself. This tension may make the client feel as if his weight control program is a failure and so he may give up and eat even more. Instead, the client should consider this as a *setback* not a failure and promise himself to do better at the next meal.

Continual distress, insomnia, headaches, fatigue, or indigestion may be danger signals of stress. Goals that are detrimental to you physically, mentally, or emotionally are not worth striving to accomplish. If your goals are too demanding, change them so they are more realistic for a healthy lifestyle.

Do something that interests you on a non-competitive level. There are hundreds of hobbies or recreations to choose from. If you find you are worrying too much, intense absorption in a hobby will help you focus your mind on other things for awhile. Try to find a hobby that really interests you. You won't experience the pleasure of accomplishment unless you try it.

So many things in life are free: parks, museums, sports, gardens, libraries, beaches, lakes, mountains—the sights, sounds, and smells of nature. Use your senses to see, hear, feel, taste, and smell the world around you. Remember, you only have one chance to live this day, so live it wisely.

Successful people (whether economically, spiritually, emotionally, socially, physically, or intellectually) are those who know that by getting up after a fall and persevering they can learn from the tough times and make their own breaks in life. They can ensure their own success. This "never give up" attitude enables many people who encounter problems to look for and find solutions. Successful people are persistent people.

Positive Imaging

Positive imaging is a mental activity in which you vividly picture in your mind a desired goal or dream and hold that image until it sinks into your subconscious where it releases untapped energies. These creative energies, gifts from the Creator, will give you ideas to reach your goals.

Taking control of your life and overcoming worry, failure, and other negative stumbling blocks can be difficult at times. It takes more than a positive attitude to conquer the things that stand between you and your dream. However, an image formed and held tenaciously in the conscious mind will pass, by a process of mental osmosis, into the subconscious mind. This powerful positive subconscious image will become a reality.

Imaging is positive thinking carried one step further. You don't just hope your dream will materialize. Instead, you visualize or see your dream as a reality and successful without any doubts whatsoever. Persistent imaging will allow your subconscious to accept your goal or objective. When this happens, powerful internal forces will be brought out which may bring astonishing changes in your life.

To illustrate how imaging works, I will give you a personal example. As a young boy, I was scared to death of speaking in public. Just the thought of getting up in front of people, especially my peers, made me break into a sweat. Then came that horrid day when my teacher gave us a public speaking assignment. My mouth went dry, and my heart beat rapidly at the thought of getting up in front of all those people. However, as I researched my assignment, I came upon a man named Demosthenes. It appeared as though he had the same problem as I did, but he did something about it. After suffering through a humiliating public experience, Demosthenes studied the art of speaking. Soon he became a great orator and one of the greatest public speakers ever.

When I lay down in bed at night, I could see Demosthenes standing before thousands of people, holding their attention with every word that spewed from his mouth. Eventually I saw a mental vision of myself standing in front of large crowds of people, feeling relaxed, confident, and energetic. I could see the multitudes of people moving as one body behind bright lights that blinded me. I could feel the surge of energy and enthusiasm as I walked confidently to the center of the stage with my microphone in hand.

As a teenager, in bed and just before sleep, I often imagined myself speaking before 4,200 people at the old Winnipeg Auditorium. Today I enjoy speaking to thousands of people across North America. My vision has become a reality, and I am living my dream. I became exactly what I imagined myself to be. We become what we think the most about.

On the negative side, I cannot help but think of all the people in hospitals or at home who are sick, who could feel so much better with positive imaging. If it does not work, what have you lost? At least you made a good effort. However, chances are great that people who use these techniques will feel at least a little bit better. Some will feel much better, and a number of folks will dissolve their problem like magic. Imagine if these techniques were used consistently in every hospital, school, home, and business where people want to use 100 percent of their brain power.

About 10 years ago, I was traveling in Alberta with one of my finest touring managers, Tony Hicks. One cold winter night, while loading a few things in the van, Tony slipped on the ice and cut his forehead. The cut was large enough to warrant taking him to the hospital. While we were at the hospital, the surgeon suggested that we use hypnosis as the sole anesthetic for the stitching. (Apparently, hypnosis was relatively new to the surgeon and he wanted to experiment with it during a small surgical procedure.) In addition to hypnotizing Tony for the procedure, I gave him a post-hypnotic suggestion that the injured area would remain numb for a 24-hour period, as opposed to medication which would likely wear off within the hour.

Remember the most important imagined pictures in your life are the ones you hold in your head about yourself. A detailed specific goal choice is one of the most important steps in your program. Secondly, specify in writing when you expect to reach your goal; be realistic.

Carefully work out a plan to reach your goal, including any sacrifices you must make to reach your goal. Is the goal worth the sacrifices? Consistently keep faith that you will reach your goal, and it is only a matter of time.

You must gather as much knowledge as possible that is directly related to your chosen goal. Educate yourself with practical knowledge; do research in libraries; seek the advice of others. Study how other people have been successful at attaining your chosen goal. Avoid wasting time on things that do not relate to achieving your goal. Say to yourself: "This is not getting me anywhere."

Planning is only effective if you include "action" in your plan. Too many people dream or make plans, but never put them to work. I've attended seminars where there are "information junkies." They suck up every bit of information they can, but never put it into action to help themselves or others. They feel that they never know enough. Their desire for perfection paralyzes their action.

Decisions must be made, mistakes will be made, and learning will take place to do better. Don't wait for a break. Instead, make your own break. You must work for what you want and do not expect to reach your goal without hard work. As my father always said, "Make your own good luck."

Temporary setbacks need not discourage you. Learn from them. Change your plans whenever necessary, but avoid repeatedly changing your goals. Determine what you want and go after it until you succeed but be careful what you go after, you probably will get it.

Once you have firmly decided on your goal, and your mind is made up to succeed at it, then use positive imaging. Soon you will begin to get hunches, flashes, insights, and ideas that will help you to form a plan to reach your goal. Ideas may come in the daytime or at night. Have a notebook and pen (or tape recorder) always close at hand. Record your ideas for they are quickly forgotten. These ideas come from the subconscious and often disappear like dreams, as quickly as they appear. Learn to trust your subconscious and believe these ideas will come. Free your mind to welcome these flashes of intuition.

The more work you devote to reaching your goal, the more your subconscious will work creatively for you. Trust your subconscious and act upon its revelations to help you succeed. The more trust you have in accessing your inner brain power, the more miracles you will receive from the gift within.

Cults and Hypnosis

Hypnosis is not a cult, nor is it evil or dangerous. A cult's main objective is to control its members' thoughts. On ABC News *Nightline*, cult expert Steven Hassan said, "If anyone is listening and they say, 'Oh I could never be seduced by mind control in a cult,' you are vulnerable." Cults use a variety of techniques of psychological coercion to achieve this. I will list some of these cult techniques of thought control to differentiate cults from safe positive hypnosis:

Isolation: Loss of reality induced by physical separation from society and rational references.

Change of Diet: Disorientation and increased susceptibility to emotional arousal achieved by depriving the nervous system of necessary nutrients, through the use of low-protein food.

Hypnosis: Focusing attention for high suggestibility. May be disguised by another word, such as meditation.

Metacommunication: Subliminal messages implanted by stressing certain key words or phrases in long, confusing lectures. For example, I remember the time I was speaking to an unhypnotized audience on the topic of the brain's power to create a feeling of immobility and numbness in an arm through hypnotic suggestion. Every time I said the words numb, unable to move, or stiff, I would give a glance directly into the eyes of some individual in the audience. It was not unusual for this person to develop such a dramatic feeling of weight in his arm that he temporarily was unable to move it. I would do this to show the *power of mere words*. Such is the strength of indirect waking (non-hypnosis) suggestion.

Discouraging Questions: To facilitate the automatic acceptance of new beliefs.

Denouncing of Current Values and Beliefs: To facilitate acceptance of the new beliefs of the cult.

Non-stop Chanting or Singing: Constant repetition of chants or phrases to focus attention and, thus, create a focused mental state of hyper-suggestibility, similar to hypnosis. This may involve hours and hours of repeating the same word or phrase to eliminate non-cult beliefs and also to establish cult beliefs.

Sleep Deprivation and Induced Fatigue: Created by preventing adequate rest and sleep through never-ending lectures, non-stop mental and physical activities, and senseless games. This lack of sleep disorients the mind making it vulnerable to the molding of new belief systems.

Peer Pressure: Need to belong to a group is exploited to encourage acceptance of new ideas and to eradicate old ideas.

Labeling: All outsiders are described as wrong, evil, or in league with the devil.

Evocation of Guilt or Fear: Elicitation of confessions and accusations of sinful past behavior and thoughts; loyalty to staying in the group reinforced by threats possibly as severe as corporal punishment; injury to the body or even death for the thoughts or behavior which are contrary to the group. Also, threats of being excommunicated from the group without any further contacts or the threat of the loss of eternal salvation.

Confusion Methods and No Privacy: Never-ending lectures or sermons that are incomprehensible, with no time alone to think or to create criticisms for the doctrine. Similar actions may be rewarded or punished at different times.

Clothing: Individuality is removed by having everyone wear the same clothing. In addition, members may have to adopt a certain hairstyle or shave all hair.

Games and Stimulation of Childish Behavior: Use of nonsensical games with confusing rules requiring frequent clarification and dependence.

Destruction of Old Relationships and Building New Ones: Because the outside world is said to be so evil, even contact by telephone may be prohibited. Attention, excessive praise, hugging, kissing, and touching may be a powerful tool. Members may be "assigned" other members and married. Another technique is isolation from media, family, friends, and books which may have competing ideas.

Securing the Member's Assets By Donation: With all assets given away to finance "worthy" group projects, the member becomes even more dependent upon the group.

Promise of Power and Salvation: Baits members with the promise that "you can work your way up the ladder" in the group by recruiting new members and by raising money for the "cause." You learn that you are a member of a group that supposedly has exclusive rights to eternal salvation.

These techniques are not used by all cults, nor are they necessarily evil. Many of these techniques are used in the military as well. However, the power of these tools has been used in a destructive manner by cults to entrap and to coercively persuade. This has resulted in the destruction of personal freedom of individual thoughts, feelings, and choices. The end result is mind control and replacement of old thoughts, beliefs, and feelings with those of the cult.

Members can be controlled to such an extent that they will do anything to please their leader, including bizarre murder. Jeannie Mills, a survivor of the Jonestown massacre in Guyana, said, "When you meet the friendliest people you have ever known, who introduce you to the most loving group of people you've ever encountered, and you find the leader to be the most inspired, caring, compassionate, and understanding person you've ever met, and then you learn that the cause of the group is something you never dared hope could be accomplished, and all of this sounds too good to be true—it probably is too good to be true! Don't give up your education, your hopes, and your ambitions to follow a rainbow."

CAUTION: *Be careful of accepting invitations by strangers to free meals, "parties" and "let's work together to help humanity causes," especially those located in remote areas, where you may not have transportation to leave.*

Positive hypnosis, such as I practice, does not take over your thoughts, values, or ideals. I oppose the use of hypnosis for anything except for positive applications, and I do not believe in controlling people's thoughts. However, I do teach people to take control of their own mind and life, in a way that they feel best helps them to reach their own goals.

If you have any doubts regarding a hypnotherapist's qualifications, I suggest that you research his or her membership status in legitimate professional organizations, that you find out the extent of his training and where he trained, and that you discuss the use of hypnosis with your own physician. If the hypnotist seems a little hostile, secretive, or nervous while you are inquiring about his qualifications, I suggest that you look elsewhere. A true professional considers questions concerning his qualifications to be quite acceptable.

10

Brain Power Exercises

This section of the book will teach you to program positive thoughts and images into your subconscious mind so that you will be able to achieve your goals quickly and efficiently.

You will learn how to enter the brain power (BP) state of mind. The BP state is calm, peaceful, and relaxed. References to sleep will be made, but you will not fall asleep. In the BP state, you will notice that three things will happen. First, you will become relaxed. Your legs, arms, and entire body may feel very heavy. You may feel sleepy and tired.

Secondly, as your body relaxes, you will find your mind concentrating and focusing almost exclusively on your own inner thoughts and self-suggestions. They will seem to completely dominate your field of attention. You will be aware of everything around you, but any sounds will simply take on a role as background to your concentration. Finally, because of your relaxed mind and body and your concentration on your self-suggestions, you will find that it should be easy to be successful with these exercises.

Begin by sitting in your favorite chair or lying on the chesterfield or bed. If you are sitting, place your feet flat on the floor and rest your hands loosely in your lap or by your side. Loosen any tight clothing that you might be wearing so that you can breathe freely and easily.

Avoid crossing your arms and legs as this creates tension. The goal is relaxation, to allow all tension to disappear and to let relaxation take its place. Adjust yourself to feel totally comfortable.

You may wish to record the following:

"You are about to experience a very pleasant state of mind. Remember, you won't be asleep; you will be conscious of everything around you. However, you will find it increasingly easier to concentrate upon your self-suggestions. There is no need to concentrate hard. Some people possess the ability to summon the BP almost immediately, while others have to develop it. With your 100 percent cooperation, you will master this skill easily.

"Now close your eyes. Inhale four deep breaths slowly and smoothly. (Pause) Think only of sleep. Deep relaxing sleep. Imagine your arms are heavy, very heavy. Imagine your legs are growing heavy, incredibly heavy. Imagine your *entire body* is heavy.

"You are relaxing more and more. Your eyes are closed. Your head is heavy. Your eyelids feel heavy like lead. Very tired. Entering the relaxed, restful world of Brain Power Consciousness. You are effortlessly focusing your concentration. A world of sleepiness, heaviness, and relaxation.

"In a few seconds, you will open your eyes and choose a bright spot, any spot, that captures your attention. You will concentrate upon that bright spot. I will soon begin counting from 20 to 1. When I say each *even* number, I would like you to *open* your eyes and stare at that one spot. When I say each *odd* number, you will then *close* your eyes and think about relaxing your mind and body. Even when your eyes are closed, you will keep staring at the spot as though you are looking right through your closed eyelids.

"With every count, you will imagine that you are relaxing deeper and deeper. With every count you, will feel more and more tired. By the time I reach the count of one, your eyelids will feel very heavy.

"**20:** open your eyes and find a spot, any spot you prefer, and keep your eyes upon it. As you watch that spot you will feel your eyelids growing heavier and heavier. It will be harder and harder to keep them open. Allow the heaviness of your eyes to make you want to close them. Let them close at the next number or before. When they are closed, keep staring at the spot through your eyelids as though you can see through your closed eyelids.

"**19:** staring and closing. **18:** watching that spot. **17:** eyelids growing heavier and heavier. **16:** relax, relax, relax. **15:** entering the deep, relaxing, restful world of sleep, a world of sleepiness, heaviness, tiredness, and beautiful relaxation. **14:** heavy head, eyelids like lead, going deeper and deeper relaxed. **13:** breathing deep and free—deep and free—breathing smoothly and easily—regularly and freely. **12:** relaxing more and more. **11:** half relaxed—your legs are growing heavy—very heavy. **10:**... **9:** your arms are growing heavy—very heavy. **8:**... **7:** your entire body is growing heavy—very heavy. **6:**... **5:** your legs are heavy—your arms are heavy—your entire body is heavy. **4:** your eyes are so tired; you feel so tired. **3:** going down, down, down, deeper and deeper and deeper to relaxation and sleep. **2:** relax deeper and deeper and deeper—tired—tired—tired so drowsy and sleepy. **1:** (pause) your eyes are closing and you are so very relaxed and everything seems to be drifting farther and farther away—sinking down, down, down—deeper and deeper to relaxation—relax, relax, relax, only sleep, sleep, sleep."

You probably will find that when you say "*you* are experiencing a sensation," it is best used if you are being hypnotized by someone else. Also, if you are making a recording to hypnotize yourself, "*you*" will likely have stronger results than "*I* am experiencing this or that." A recording will help you to relax and focus your energies more efficiently because all you need to do is simply listen.

However, if you are giving yourself mental suggestions, then using the word "*I*" at the start of each self-suggestion likely will bring you the greatest success. Another tip: Be sure to *allow* your eyelids to feel heavier and heavier as the numbers are spoken from 20 to 1. Continue your recorded suggestions as follows:

"Your body and mind are now relaxed. Your mind is in a receptive mental state—the BP state—receptive to suggestions for reaching your goals successfully. With your mind so concentrated, you will find that you want to follow your own positive suggestions."

With practice you will be able to attain a deeper and deeper BP state. Generally, the more deeply you enter the state, the more susceptible you are to the suggestions you give yourself. For example, pain control is more effective with a *deeper* hypnotic state. You may then influence your subconscious mind, that part that controls your waking and sleeping life. Soon you will be able to use this newly developed skill quickly and naturally anywhere, anytime.

Mind Calming

It may help to be alone in a room unless others are also planning to enjoy the experience as well. Most people prefer the room to be dark or darker than usual, although this is not necessary. The room should be relatively quiet, especially if you are a beginner. Comfort is most important, so sit in your favorite chair or lie down upon a comfortable couch.

Once you are comfortable, inhale and exhale three or four deep breaths. Breathe out slowly. Breathe in through your nose and breathe out through your mouth. Your lips should always be parted slightly to assist your facial muscles in relaxing. A relaxed face and slightly open mouth are good facilitators and indicators of hypnosis.

With your eyes half open, find a spot, line, or anything that captures your attention. Stare at it in a relaxed and dreamy way. Unless you resist, your eyelids will feel heavy and will want to close lightly, but not tightly. *Relax your eyelids so much that they feel too heavy to open.* (If you are reading this, you can just let yourself drift into a nice trance. Sink deeper into relaxation with every word that you see with your eyes. You can come out of this trance by simply counting from one to five, by thinking or saying the numbers aloud.)

Now turn your thoughts to various parts of your body. Imagine the separate parts growing heavy. As you think of each part of your body, become aware of any tension or tightness in that part of your body and let it go.

Start with your feet. Notice the tightness in the muscles, the toes, and the heels. Let them go and completely relax. Imagine your feet going numb, temporarily. Remember the feeling when you awakened in the middle of the night and your arm had felt numb from sleeping on it. Or, recreate the feeling you had when the dentist injected chemicals to anesthetize your jaw to make it feel numb. Imagine in terms of feelings and pictures rather than words which are hollow and have less emotional impact.

Once your feet feel like dead weights, relax your calves, knees, back of your knees, hips, thighs, waist, and stomach muscles. Make sure your lips are still parted and that your facial muscles are relaxed. Relax your chest, the lower part of your back at your waist, your middle back, and the upper part of your back.

Now let your shoulders droop and hang loosely. Think of relaxing the muscles in your throat, your mouth, and your tongue—even the nerves in your teeth. Then relax your lips, your jaw, your cheeks, and your eyes. Let all the wrinkles in your forehead smooth away. Now relax the back of your head, the nape of your neck, and finally the scalp. There is no need to memorize the above in order. Just relax the body and mind step by step from the bottom of your feet to the top of your head.

After becoming totally relaxed, let your mind *ponder* the specific changes you want to occur in your personality or habits. See yourself going through your daily life as the person you want to be, doing the things you want to do. The application of BP is just that simple.

With repetition, these positive thought pictures automatically are filtered through to your unconscious mind. You will start to find yourself spontaneously doing the things that you want to do; feeling the way you want to feel; becoming more cheerful, positive, and optimistic.

The more senses these positive "daydreams" use, the more permanent the effect. The more vivid and lifelike you allow these daydreams to become, the better. Write down in detail what you plan to imagine in hypnosis before you actually begin your session. This way you will not have to be disturbed by trying to create suggestions while you are in the BP state. Be realistic and, in time, you will follow your self-suggestions automatically.

If you want to improve your study habits or concentration skills, visualize yourself with perfect concentration. Imagine that minor sounds or distractions do not disturb you. See, in your imagination, your textbook in your hand and the chair on which you are seated. Feel, in your imagination, the cover of the book and the straight back of the chair. Imagine yourself fascinated with the book and absorbing the information you are reading. However, do not suggest to yourself that you will have a 100 percent perfect photographic memory as this is unrealistic. This would only lead to a feeling of disappointment and discouragement.

Other imagined "stories" or scenes may involve recall. Imagine yourself easily remembering facts and information with answers flowing freely through your mind, both in the classroom and during examinations. Improvements usually will be gradual and progressive. With concentration, for example, you probably will experience noticeable improvement after just a few sessions. Occasionally, "miracles" occur within a short time.

After a number of sessions, you should notice that you can relax mentally and physically within a few seconds. You can then spend most of the session imagining successful scenes. You should be able to relax quickly because you have developed a *memory pattern*. A memory pattern is a chain of responses or "hooked" thoughts. Some people train themselves to relax from the bottom of their feet to the top of their head by merely thinking of the word "calm" or "relax." Some people take more than a few sessions to learn how to relax. If you rush relaxation during your early training, you will only obtain its opposite effect—tension! Some people record their hypnotic induction on tape and listen to it, without need for any conscious effort. I suggest that you do this. Sometimes, having one's own voice giving the hypnotic suggestions may be the most effective.

I encourage you to try different approaches such as variations in your recorded voice, perhaps using the voice of someone else, and with and without music

Accessing the Brain Power State Quickly

When you are in hypnosis, feeling deeply relaxed, give yourself a *post-hypnotic suggestion* that the next time you wish to enter the brain power state of relaxation, all you have to do is make a tight fist with your right hand. Tell yourself that as you notice the tightness in your fingers, the back of the hand, the wrist and the muscles, you will relax. Simply tell yourself that as you relax that hand, you will allow the relaxation to *flow* to your right arm, shoulders, left arm, upper body, mid-section, and lower body—thus, relaxing you all over in seconds. Tell yourself that you are going into a deeper and deeper relaxation with each and every breath.

Imagination Exercise

You must learn to use your power of imagination in order to achieve control of your mind and body. Mind control is a mental discipline enabling you to influence your thoughts, feelings, and behavior. By mastering the exercises described in this book, you gradually will gain remarkable control over the personal habits you wish to influence.

The following text will help you develop this skill of mental mastery. Like any other skill, practice is important in order to respond positively. Your BP training should be done in the privacy of your home. It is helpful to avoid excessive noise or distractions. You also may suggest to yourself: "These sounds or distractions, unless an emergency, send me deeper and deeper into hypnosis."

Once your are successful with several of these tests, you will have developed greater confidence in your ability to go into hypnosis rapidly. You also will feel confident about being able to follow any positive hypnotic suggestion to enhance your life. These experiments are important because they will help you to develop the skill of following hypnotic suggestions rapidly:

Experiment #1

Close your eyes and suggest the following in your own words, "In a few seconds I will begin to feel a tickling sensation in my throat, a need and desire to swallow. This urge will become so incredibly intense I will have to swallow to have relief. As this urge intensifies, I find it most interesting. I will satisfy it; I will swallow."

Experiment #2

Stand tall, but relaxed, with your feet together and your arms raised forward and upward until they are outstretched before you. Visualize your arms and hands in front of you with your eyes closed.

Now picture your right arm beginning to rise and your left arm starting to fall. Picture the right arm rising higher while your left arm falls lower. It may help if you imagine a balloon filled with helium attached to your right arm and also imagine your left arm weighted down with a pail of sand.

Experiment #3

Stretch your arms out in front of you. Clasp your hands together. Tell yourself that your hands are the jaws of a vise, gripping and frozen together. Imagine the vise is tightening and the jaws (your hands) are locked. Your eyes should be closed. Closing your eyes helps your mind to use a more vivid imagination since there are no visual distractions.

Just squeeze your hands together, mentally thinking, "My hands are sticking, locking, freezing, gluing, cementing tighter and tighter together. At the count of three, I cannot release them. The harder I try, the tighter they stick." Then tell yourself that you can release them when you say aloud the word "release" three times. Again, this could be recorded, changing the word "I" to "you."

Experiment #4

Sit in a chair and imagine you are stuck and cannot get up. Think rapidly over and over, "I am stuck, glued, completely stuck." Then release yourself by saying aloud the word "release" three times.

Experiment #5

Imagine a certain part of your body is itchy and that you must scratch it.

Experiment #6

Press the tips of two of your fingers together and imagine the tips of your fingers are locked together. Or, press your middle finger and thumb together and push. Stare at them while telling yourself a strong glue is binding them together. Tell yourself that nothing can separate your fingers until you reverse the suggestion by imagining that they are now unglued.

Experiment #7

Imagine a powerful bonding glue pouring around your eyelids. Imagine your eyelids are glued together.

Experiment #8

Imagine that your right foot is so heavy that it cannot move. Imagine that you cannot lift your right foot off the ground until you, and only you, decide to release that suggestion.

Experiment #9

Stiffen your right arm and imagine that it is a rigid bar of steel. Imagine that you cannot bend your right arm until you wish to do so.

Experiment #10

Shake your hands in front of you (a method of relaxation in itself). Imagine you cannot stop shaking them until you wish to do so. You might mentally think: "My hands are shaking faster and faster, going out of control. Faster and faster. Out of control." Then you might release with, "I can now stop my hands from shaking. My hands stop and I relax them."

Experiment #11

Open your mouth and imagine that you cannot close it. Or close it and imagine that you cannot open it, until you decide you want to.

You may not achieve positive results with all the previous tests until you become familiar with the deeper levels of self-hypnosis.

The more you develop your imagination through practice, the more susceptible you will be to hypnosis and the deeper the hypnotic state you will be able to achieve. As a result, you also will be more delighted with your success!

Those few people experiencing great obstacles in this area of instruction should take advantage of recordings made by hypnotists. If you need additional help, contact a professional hypnotist for personal instruction. The road to success is open to virtually anyone, although some may take a little more time than others. I often say at my seminars, "Fast or slow, it doesn't matter, we all learn how to do it."

Imaging Exercise

This imaging technique may be helpful if a stubborn problem is harassing or troubling you. Take 30 seconds right now and picture yourself taking command over that problem. See yourself solving it, overcoming it, moving beyond it into a realm of confidence where other problems will be met and overcome as they arise.

Then take three long deep breaths and exhale slowly after each one.

As you take the first one, say to yourself, "I'm breathing in confidence; I'm breathing out tension."

With the second and third: "I'm *breathing in* victory and success over my problem of (name it); I'm *breathing out* tension."

Visualize new confidence and enthusiasm flowing into you. You can take control of your life.

Key Beneficial Suggestions During Brain Power Sessions

1. Instill feelings of relaxation, safety, and security.
2. Instill forgiveness for yourself and others.
3. Build up your confidence.
4. Instill feelings of self-control and empowerment.
5. Instill a feeling of strong will power.
6. Instill a feeling that you have choices and alternative modes of response. In other words, develop an automatic response such that if what you are doing is not working, then you easily switch to another method. There is no need to keep pushing an immovable obstacle; just try another route to succeed. As the saying goes: "Why bang your head against a wall?" There are usually many

highways leading to the same destination of happiness and success.

More About Brain Power Training

Try to enjoy at least one brain power training period each 24-hour period. When you go to bed, assume the same position you usually do when you sleep at night. When you sense you are about to fall asleep, begin suggesting to yourself ideas such as the following: "My legs feel heavy, very heavy. My arms feel heavy, very heavy. My entire body is heavy—heavy with relaxation and tiredness." (It is not necessary to memorize any suggestions: just give yourself similar suggestions in your own words.)

"In the future, whenever I wish to focus my mind in the relaxed brain power state, all I need do is sit down or lie down, close my eyes and slowly take in four deep breaths. I will feel completely relaxed with the fourth breath. Each time that I breathe in, I will imagine the lower, middle, or upper part of my body relaxing. On the first breath out, I relax the lower part of my body. On the second breath out, I relax the middle part of my body. On the third breath, I relax the upper part of my body. On the fourth breath, I will relax my mind. I relax more with each additional breath."

Give yourself the above suggestions each night. You should induce relatively deep levels of mental focusing in less than 30 days. Again, if you have any difficulties, you should use a hypnotic recording or consult a competent hypnotist to aid you.

Coming Out of the Brain Power State of Mind

To come out of the brain power state of mind, simply suggest to yourself, "At the count of five, I will come back to the room feeling happy, relaxed, and alert having enjoyed my rest. At five, I *instantly* will feel sound in body, sound in mind, sound in spirit, and sound in health.

"**1:** I am slowly awakening. (Picture and feel yourself full of energy and enthusiasm as you do this.) **2:** I am almost awake. My body feels a surge of energy, relaxation, and confidence. **3:** My thinking is crystal clear. **4:** I am opening my eyes. **5:** I am wide awake! Feeling fantastic!"

Here is another example of a "coming out" script: "At the count of five, you will wiggle your toes, stretch, and then inhale a deep breath while thinking about how you feel *successful* and *in control* of your life." The word "you" may be changed to "I," if you are doing self-hypnosis.

Feel free to try variations of the procedure described above. You may invent one that is far more effective for your needs. Each person is so unique that programs may be greatly individualized.

Remember to *build up your powers of visualization* and to imagine actual scenarios that you would like to happen. The more vivid your visualization, the more powerful will be your auto-suggestions. And most wonderful of all is the never-ending realization that the more you practice, the better you will become at using this incredible inborn skill, tapped by so few people.

For example, close your eyes and relax your body and mind. Then, vividly imagine yourself remaining calm in a pressure situation. We become our thoughts. Continue your studies of the mind with audio and video recordings, books, and seminars.

Best of all, this gift of the Creator is free. Since no one talks to you as much as you do, be sure your "talk" is more positive each day.

Most people do not make use of this gift, because they do not know it is there or refuse to believe it is there. If you believe—it is so! You are your own hypnotist and what you think about, you become. Your thoughts influence every cell of your brain and body. Use your powers to create a heaven of health and happiness for yourself and others.

Many years ago, psychologist Sidney M. Jourard wrote in his book, *The Transparent Self,* about how constantly hiding our real self with various masks brings ill health. Dr. Jourard says: "...failure or inability to know and be one's real self can make one sick... Authentic being means being oneself, honestly... dropping pretense, defenses, and duplicity... while simple honesty with others (and thus to oneself) may yield scars, it is likely to be an effective preventive both of mental illness and of certain kinds of physical sickness. Honesty can literally be a health-insurance policy."

11

Conclusion

In this book I quoted Napoleon as saying, "Imagination rules the world." We must certainly agree that our imagination rules our lives. You have learned that your subconscious can be your master or your *servant*. Successful people, people in control of their lives, have learned to master and control the subconscious forces of their mind. Thus, your subconscious mind becomes your servant. On a daily basis, as often as possible, it is a good idea to decide to deliberately program positive success images into your inner mind. I did not say words. I said images. It has been said a picture is worth a thousand words, and if your success "picture" holds *emotional intensity* or powerful feelings, the strength is greatly multiplied.

Many years ago, Anton Mesmer was denounced as a fraud because the commission who investigated his thousands of successful cures attributed his healing powers to the mere imagination of his patients. When I was a teenager, a young man wanted me to hypnotize him. I handed him a bottle of placebo pills which should have had no effect whatsoever. I told him the bottle contained hypnotics, as I had neatly typed the word "hypnotics" on the label. He swallowed one pill and within one minute he was in a deep hypnotic trance. The pills were bogus, and hypnosis was induced by his own mind. *What a dramatic example of the powers of the imagination!*

When you enter your brain power state of consciousness called trance or hypnosis, all you have to say is: "Unconscious, with all your brilliance and kindness, please instruct me how I may lose weight permanently; how I may quit smoking permanently; how I may improve my memory; etc."

Your unconscious mind will deliver the exact unique individual answer to you to help solve your problem. This answer may come in the trance, in a dream, walking down the street, while relaxing in a warm bath, or at some other time, quite by surprise. It cannot be said exactly how or when your unconscious will solve the problem, but it will. As you would respect any great creative genius, have great respect for the inner you, your unconscious mind. Always thank your unconscious for its work to solve the problem. Again, gratefully thank your unconscious when it gives you the solution.

Some will say, "This will not possibly work," but they will lose this great gift from the Creator. It is known that if one believes a voodoo curse can kill him, he is likely to imagine and enlarge the power of the witch doctor in his mind. Being terrified, he may die of a heart attack. However, if one is unaware of the so-called "witch doctor's curse," nothing happens. Imagination may keep us a prisoner to worry about the impending future or may create mental barriers capping our potential. Conversely, the right imagined thoughts may release positive chemicals within our body to heal us and carry us toward our visions of success, health, and happiness.

In September 1994, I read a related story in *The Now Newspaper* distributed in Burnaby, British Columbia. The write-up was about a family who lived next door to a neighbor who claimed he was Lucifer. In 1991, this neighbor claimed that he had put a curse on the father. In 1993, the couple became increasingly worried because their daughter was having seizures and, subsequently, became convinced that an evil force was overpowering them. The couple believed that their daughter's cradle rocked by itself. The cradle was then burned to exorcise the spirit. The wife had visualizations and nightmares that their baby was being taken out of the bedroom by a supernatural force or evil spirit. This all ended with the father, his wife, and daughter driving their vehicle into a concrete pillar, killing all three of them. They *believed* that they were cursed by Satan. Such are the dangers of wrong imagined thoughts.

The curve of success is never straight with brain power mental focusing. Sometimes you will have set-backs and at other times spectacular successes. In this journey of adventure into your mind, your greatest successes will come with knowledge and practice. Combine this with a belief in yourself and the BP method and you will maximize the development of these superior skills. There is no end to the learning, and there is no limit to the possibilities of your imagination. Believe, and it is so.

I would like to end with one of my favorite stories, which I first heard from Dr. William J. Bryan, Jr. A ferocious tiger chased a man to the edge of a cliff. The man jumped off the edge and was able to grasp a branch. Unfortunately, another tiger was waiting for him at the bottom of the cliff and the branch was breaking. At that point, he picked one of the brightly colored cherries growing on the branch and began eating it.

Forgetting about the terror above and below him, he said, "What a delicious fruit." Consider that this precious day will never be again. Enjoy every moment!

In June 1996, a personal tragedy occurred in my life involving my own family. This was the most stressful event that has ever occurred in my life. In this time of stress, I lost 15 pounds in three weeks. I received support from many sources including my mother, my father, my brother, my friends, relatives, the Catholic Church, and books. To my delight, one of the greatest supports that renewed my personal strength actually came to me by reading my own book, the one you have in your hand.

I realized that focusing on the past—that which cannot be changed—left me helpless. If I were to blame anyone, I would only feel like a victim. For my own benefit, it became a necessity to forgive. I had to accept that I could not control other people's choices. However, I could control my own behavior and my own thoughts and reactions to their choices.

Why fight and struggle to change what cannot be changed? I had to focus on the present and on the future, where I will spend the rest of my life. Instead of saying, "Why did this happen to us?" I had to say, "What can I do about it now? How can I apply my God-given intelligence and strengths to make our lives happier?" My thoughts could change me from being a victim to being victorious.

Let me leave you with two quotations, the origin of which I am unaware. My mother sent these words to me during this most painful time of my life: "Winners are like tea bags. You never see their strength until they are in hot water." "Our greatest glory consists not in never falling, but in rising every time we fall."

Romane Self-Help, Home-Use Programs

Romane Hypnosis Cassettes

Only $20.00 each. *Warning: Do Not Play Hypnosis Audio-Cassette Recordings while Driving.*

1. Enjoy Dental Visits with No Fear and No Pain. Romane had a tooth pulled in self-hypnosis, with no anesthetic. He felt nothing when the tooth was pulled.
2. Positive Mental Attitude and Confidence at Job Interviews. For those seeking employment.
3. Side A: Improve Memory. Side B: Be Motivated to Study.
4. Side A: Be Motivated to Do and Enjoy Exercise. Side B: Enjoy Good Health.
5. Side A: Have Fun Experiencing Past Lives. Side B: Astral Energizing—Take a Trip without the Ticket.
6. Side A: End Procrastination. Side B: Replace Fear of Failure with Expectation of Success.
7. Side A: Develop Powerful Concentration. Side B: Be Relaxed and Have a Great Memory During Examinations.
8. Side A: Cut Down or Stop Drinking Alcohol. Side B: End Sexual Impotence.
9. Side A: Better Golfing with Imagery and Hypnosis. Side B: Better Bowling.
10. Side A: Fall Asleep and Awaken Refreshed. Side B: Banish Worry.
11. Side A: Enjoy Doing Housework. Side B: Use the Power of Colors and Visual Imagery to Change Your Life.
12. Side A: Be a Great Conversationalist. Side B: Make Friends Easily.
13. Side A: Stop Nail Biting for Attractive Hands. Side B: Be Confident, Enhance Self-Esteem, and Be More Assertive.
14. Side A: Increase Your Energy and Enthusiasm. Side B: Best of Health.
15. Side A: Banish Negative Images and Memories of the Past. Side B: Achieve Your Maximum Happiness.

16. Side A: How to Develop a Money Magnet Mind for Prosperity. Side B: Program Your Mind for Success.
17. For Women: Love Your Body. Enhance Self-Esteem.
18. Side A: Secrets of Creativity. Side B: Be a Successful Problem Solver.
19. Side A: Stop Stuttering and Speak Confidently. Side B: Be a Dynamic Public Speaker.
20. Develop Your Sensory Imagery for Better Imagery and Faster Success.
21. Side A: Banish Jealousy. Side B: Be Forgiving to Yourself and Others for Your Benefit.
22. Side A: How to Reach Your Goals. Side B: Develop Enthusiasm.
23. Eliminate Tension Headaches with Any of These Methods.
24. Perfection in Piano. Play your best and be relaxed during exams, recitals, and performances.

Music for Relaxation, Meditation, Massage, and Peace of Mind

25. Side A: Astral Violet by Sondra Gordon. Side B: Past, Present, Future by Christopher Lee Pavlik.
26. Side A: Ocean Sounds by Tony Scrace. Side B: Journey Within by Tony Scrace.

Cassette Audio Tape Sets

1. Weight Loss Seminar

Two cassettes running about two hours with a complete seminar recorded live, plus a third tape for reinforcement and weight maintenance. $60.00

2. Stop Smoking Seminar

Three cassettes running about two hours with a complete seminar recorded live, plus a fourth tape for reinforcement to keep you a permanent non-smoker. The very best program! $80.00

3. Self-Hypnosis Seminar

Learn about hypnosis and why it works. Master self-hypnosis by being given post-hypnotic suggestions while you are in hypnosis. Learn how to give yourself hypnotic suggestions to overcome unhealthy habits and to achieve your maximum personal best. Three cassettes running about three hours, including confidence building cassette, and printed material. $60.00

4. Relieve Stress Seminar

   Three cassettes of a seminar running over two hours. Life has constant invitations to stress, the unseen killer. Enjoy peace of mind, be calm and be relaxed with over 20 methods. Overcome needless worry, sleep better, and enjoy the best of health in mind and body. Incudes a fourth "reinforcer" cassette. $80.00

5. Romane VHS Videotape: Stop Smoking with Hypnosis

   A revolving spiral creates a feeling of being drawn into a "tunnel". You will receive hypnotic suggestions to overcome withdrawal, cravings, irritability, and weight gain. Highly effective. Come out of hypnosis feeling relaxed and refreshed. Cameramen found themselves going into hypnosis while just filming this program. For use with the audio tapes above, or as a reinforcer if you have already taken the live seminar. $30.00

Books

The Wellness Journey (160 pages) $15.00

To Order

Please list titles desired adding $4.00 shipping for the first item and $0.75 for each additional item. Please also add applicable sales taxes. To order or to contact Romane for speaking engagements, seminars, or concerts write:

M. Vance Romane c/o M.V.P. Ltd.
Box 75177
White Rock, British Columbia
Canada V4A 9N4

Phone: 1-800-665-4656 Fax: (604) 538-8477
Email: vance@direct.ca

P.S. You are invited to send your brain power experiences to M. Vance Romane. If he includes your letter in his next book, he will send you a free autographed gift copy with your story.

Bibliography and References

Adams, Paul. *The New Self-Hypnosis*. Hollywood: Wilshire Book Company, 1975.

Alman, Vance M., and Lambrou, Peter. *Self-Hypnosis: The Complete Manual For Health and Self-Change*. New York: Brunner/Mazel, Publishers, 1992.

Araoz, Daniel L. *The New Hypnosis*. New York: Brunner/Mazel Inc., 1985.

Araoz, Daniel L., and Bleck, Robert T. *Hypnosex, Sexual Joy Through Self-Hypnosis*. New York: Arbor House, 1982.

Arluck, Edward Wiltcher. *Hypnoanalysis: A Case Study*. New York: Random House, 1964.

Arons, Harry. *Hypnosis in Criminal Investigation*. South Orange: Power Publishers, Inc., 1977.

Arons, Harry. *Handbook of Self-Hypnosis*. Irvington: Power Publishers, 1969.

Bandler, Richard, and Grinder, John. *Patterns of the Hypnotic Techniques of Milton H. Erickson, M.D.* Cupertino: Meta Publications, 1975.

Barabasz, Arreed F. *New Techniques in Behavior Therapy and Hypnosis*. South Orange: Power Publishers, Inc., 1977.

Bernstein, Morey. *The Search for Bridey Murphy*. Garden City: Doubleday & Company Inc., 1956.

Block, Eugene B. *Hypnosis: A New Tool In Crime Detection*. New York: David McKay Co., 1976.

Bowers, Kenneth S. *Hypnosis for the Seriously Curious*, New York/London: W. W. Norton & Company, 1976.

Boyne, Gil. *How to Teach Self-Hypnosis*. Robert S. Fraser, Editor, 1987.

Boyne, Gil. Hypnosis: *New Tool in Nursing Practice*. Glendale: Westwood Publishing Company, 1982.

Bristol, Claude M. *The Magic of Believing*. New York: Pocket Books, 1972.

Brooks, C. H. *Self Mastery Through Conscious Auto-Suggestion by Emile Coué & the Practice of Auto-Suggestion by the Method of Emile Coué*. London: George Allen & Unwin, 1984.

Bryan, William J., Jr., M.D. *The Chosen Ones*. Los Angeles: Westwood Publishing Co., 1971.

Caprio, Frank S., and Berger, Joseph R. *Helping Yourself with Self-Hypnosis*. New York: Warner Paperback Library, 1975.

Carnegie, Dale. *How to Win Friends and Influence People*. New York: Simon & Schuster Inc., 1981.

Carnegie, Dale. *The Dale Carnegie Course in Effective Speaking and Human Relations*. Garden City: Dale Carnegie & Associates, Inc., 1981.

Cheek, David B., M.D., and LeCron, Leslie M. *Clinical Hypnotherapy*. New York: Grune & Stratton, Inc., 1968.

Chertok, L. *Hypnosis*. Toronto: Pergamon Press, 1966.

Clarke, Christopher, and Jackson, J. Arthur. *Hypnosis and Behavior Therapy*. New York: Springer Publishing Company, Inc., 1983.

Cohen, Sherry Suib. *The Magic of Touch*. New York: Harper & Row, Publishers, 1988.

Cooke, C. E. and Van Vogt, A. E. *Hypnotism Handbook*. Alhambra: Borden Publishing Co., 1965.

Cossman, E. J., and Cohen, William A. *Making It!* Englewood Cliffs: Prentice Hall, 1994.

Coué, Emile. *How to Practice Suggestion and Auto-Suggestion*. New York: American Library Service, 1923.

Crasilneck, H. B., and Hall, J. A. *Clinical Hypnosis Principlel and Applications*. New York: Grune and Stratton, 1975.

Cunningham, Les. *Hypnosport*. Glendale: Westwood Publishing Co., 1981.

Dorcus, Roy M. *Hypnosis and Its Therapeutic Applications*. Toronto: McGraw-Hill Book Company, Inc., 1956.

Dowd, E. Thomas, and Healy, James M. *Case Studies in Hypnotherapy*. New York: The Guilford Press, 1986.

Duckworth, John. *How to Use Auto-Suggestion Effectively*. Hollywood: Wilshire Book Company, 1976.

Edmunds, Simeon. *The Psychic Power of Hypnosis*. London: The Aquarian Publishing Co. Ltd., 1978.

Eisenberg, Howard. *Inner Spaces: Parapsychological Explorations of the Mind*. Don Mills: Musson Book Company, 1977.

Ellen, Arthur. *The Intimate Casebook of a Hypnotist*. Toronto: The New American Library of Canada Limited, 1968.

Ellis, Albert, and Harper, Robert. *A Guide to Successful Marriage*. North Hollywood: Wilshire Book Company, 1977.

Elman, Dave. *Hypnotherapy*. Los Angeles: Westwood Publishing Co., 1964.

Erickson, Milton H. *Advanced Techniques of Hypnosis and Therapy*. New York: Grune & Stratton Inc., 1967.

Erickson, Milton H. *A Teaching Seminar*. New York: Brunner/Mazel, Publishers, 1980.

Erickson, Milton H. *Experiencing Hypnosis—Therapeutic Approaches to Altered States*. New York: Irvington Publishers, Inc., 1981.

Erickson, Milton H. *Hypnotic Realities*. New York: Irvington Publishers, Inc., 1976.

Erickson, Milton H. *Innovative Hypnotherapy. Volumes 1, 2, 3, & 4*. New York: Irving Publishers, Inc., 1980.

Erickson, Milton H. *My Voice Will Go with You*. New York: Norton & Company, 1982.

Erickson, Milton H.; Hershman, Seymour; and Secter, Irving I. *Medical And Dental Hypnosis*. New York: The Julian Press, Inc., 1961.

Fross, Garland H. *Handbook of Hypnotic Techniques with Special Reference to Dentistry*. South Orange: Power Publishers, Inc., 1974.

Furst, Arnold. *A Brief Course in... Hypnosis for Salesmen*. Alhambra: Borden Publishing Company, 1960.

Gardner, Gail G., and Olness, Karen, M.D. *Hypnosis and Hypnotherapy with Children*. New York: Grune and Stratton, Inc., 1981.

Gendlin, Eugene T. *Focusing*. Toronto: Bantam Books, Inc., 1981.

Gibson, Walter. *Hypnotism Theory and Practice*. Toronto: Coles Publishing Company, 1979.

Gibson, Walter. *Hypnotism Through The Ages*. New York: Vista House Publishers, 1961.

Gibson, Walter. *The Key to Hypnotism*. Baltimore: Ottenheimer Publishers, Inc., 1956.

Grouch, David A., M.D., and Fross, Garland H. *What Every Subject Should Know About Hypnosis and Self-Hypnosis*. South Orange: Power Publishers, Inc., 1976.

Gutwirth, Samuel W. *You Can Learn to Relax*. North Hollywood: Wilshire Book Company, 1974.

Hadley, Josie, and Staudacher, Carol. *Hypnosis for Change*. New York: Ballantine Books, 1987.

Haley, Jay. *Uncommon Therapy*. New York: W. W. Norton & Company, 1973.

Hart, Hornell. *Autoconditioning: The New Way to a Successful Life*. Englewood Cliffs: Prentice Hall, Inc., 1977.

Heise, Jack. *How You Can Bowl Better Using Self-Hypnosis*. Hollywood: Wilshire Book Company, 1974.

Heise, Jack. *How You Can Play Better Golf Using Self-Hypnosis*. Hollywood: Wilshire Book Company, 1974.

Heron, William T., and Hershman, Seymour, M.D. *An Old Art Returns to Medicine*. Copyright 1958.

Hilgard, Ernest R. and Josephine R. *Hypnosis in the Relief of Pain*. Los Altos: William Kaufmann, Inc., 1975.

Hoke, James H. *I Would If I Could And I Can: Program Your Personality for Success*. New York: Berkley Books, 1982.

Hollander, Bernard, M.D. *Methods and Uses of Hypnosis and Self-Hypnosis*. Hollywood: Wilshire Book Company, 1978.

Jourard, Sidney M. *The Transparent Self*. Toronto: D. Van Nostrand Company (Canada) Ltd., 1964.

Kappas, John G. *Professional Hypnotism Manual*. Panorama City: Panorama Publishing Company, 1978.

Kirtley, Christine. *Consumer Guide to Hypnosis*. Merrimack: The National Guild of Hypnotists, 1991.

Kline, Milton V. *Freud and Hypnosis: The Interaction of Psychodymanics and Hypnosis*. New York: The Julian Press, Inc., 1958.

Klippstein, Hildegard. *Ericksonian Hypnotherapeutic Group Inductions*. New York: Brunner/Mazel Publishers, 1991.

Kopp, Sheldon B. *If You Meet The Buddha On The Road, Kill Him!* New York: Bantam Books, 1981.

Kroger, William S., M.D. *Childbirth with Hypnosis*. Hollywood: Wilshire Book Company, 1961.

Kroger, William S., M.D. *Clinical and Experimental Hypnosis*. Toronto: J. B. Lippincott Company, 1977.

Kroger, William S., M.D. *Hypnosis and Behavior Modification: Imagery Conditioning*. Toronto: J. B. Lippincott Company, 1976.

Kuhns, Bradley William. *Hypnosis and The Law*. Glendale: Westwood Publishing Company, 1981.

Lankton, Stephen R. and Carol H. *The Answer Within: A Clinical Framework of Ericksonian Hypnotherapy*. New York: Brunner/Mazel, Publishers, 1983.

LeCron, Leslie M. *Self Hypnotism: The Technique and Its Use in Daily Living*. New York: The New American Library, 1964.

LeCron, Leslie M. *Techniques of Hypnotherapy*. New York: The Julian Press, 1961.

LeCron, Leslie M. *The Complete Guide to Hypnosis*. New York: Barnes and Noble Books, 1973.

Leitner, Konradi. *Successful Hypnotism For Professionals*. New York: Stravon Publishers, 1963.

Macrae, Janet. *Therapeutic Touch: A Practical Guide*. New York: Alfred A. Knopf, 1988.

Magonet, Phillip, M.D. *Practical Hypnotism*. Hollywood: Wilshire Book Company, 1976.

Marcuse, F. L. *Hypnosis Fact and Fiction*. Baltimore: Penguin Books Ltd., 1971.

McGill, Ormond. *Encyclopedia of Stage Hypnotism*. Colon: Abbott's Magic Novelty Co., 1947.

McGill, Ormond. *The Art of Stage Hypnotism*. Oakland: Magic Limited, 1975.

Morris, Freda. *Hypnosis with Friends & Lovers*. San Francisco: Harper & Row, Publishers, Inc., 1979.

Morris, Freda. *Self-Hypnosis in Two Days*. New York: E. P. Dutton & Co., Inc., 1975.

Moss, C. Scott. *Hypnosis in Perspective*. Toronto: Collier-Macmillan, 1965.

Mutke, Peter H. C., M.D. *Selective Awareness*. Millbrae: Celestial Arts, 1977.

Napowsa, Walters D. *Hypno-Technology: Roles of the Hypno-Technician*. St. Petersburg: S.O.S. Printing, 1977.

Nightingale, Earl. *The New Lead the Field*. (audiocassette album) Chicago: Nightingale-Conant Corporation, 1986.

Older, Jules. *Touching Is Healing*. New York: Stein and Day/Publishers, 1982.

Orton, Louis J. *Hypnotism Made Practical*. Hollywood: Wilshire Book Company, 1976.

Petrie, Sidney. *What Modern Hypnotism Can Do for You*. Greenwich: Fawcett Publications, Inc., 1972.

Petrie, Sidney, and Stone, Robert B. *Hypno Cybernetics. Helping Yourself to a Rich New Life*. Englewood Cliffs: Parker Publishing Company, Inc., 1976.

Powers, Melvin. *Advanced Techniques of Hypnosis*. Hollywood: Wilshire Book Company, 1978.

Powers, Melvin. *Hypnotism Revealed*. Hollywood: Wilshire Book Company, 1978.

Powers, Melvin, and Starrett, Robert S. *A Practical Guide to Better Concentration*. Hollywood: Wilshire Book Company, 1962.

Pulos, Lee. *Beyond Hypnosis*. Vancouver: Omega Press, 1990.

Rawcliffe, D. H. *Illusions and Delusions of the Supernatural and the Occult*. New York: Dover Publications, Inc., 1959.

Reardon, William T., M.D. *Modern Medical Hypnosis*. Wilmington, 1965.

Reiser, Martin. *Handbook of Investigative Hypnosis*. Los Angeles: Lehi Publishing Company, 1980.

Ringrose, C.A. Douglas, M.D. *Coping the Natural Way (Comprehensive Special Sense Therapy)*.

Schneck, Jerome M. *Hypnosis in Modern Medicine*. Springfield: Charles C. Thomas, 1963.

Segall, Martin M. *The Questions They Ask*. South Orange: Power Publishers, Inc.,1975.

Shames, Richard, M.D. and Sterin, Chuck. *Healing with Mind Power*. Emmaus: Rodale Press, 1978.

Silva, Jose. *The Silva Mind Control Method*. New York: Pocket Books, 1978.

Simonton, O. Carl, M.D. *Getting Well Again*. Los Angeles: J. P. Tarcher, Inc., 1978.

Soskis, David A. *Teaching Self-Hypnosis: An Introductory Guide for Clinicians*. New York/London: W. W. Norton & Company, 1986.

Stolzenberg, Jacob. *Psychosomatics and Suggestion Therapy in Dentistry*. New York: Philosophical Library Inc., 1950.

Straus, Roger A. *Creative Self-Hypnosis*. New York/London: Prentice Hall Press, 1989.

Tebbetts, Charles. *Self Hypnosis and Other Mind Expanding Techniques*. Glendale: Westwood Publishing Company, 1977.

Tebbetts, Charles. *Miracles on Demand: The Radical Short-Term Hypnotherapy of Gil Boyne*. Glendale: Westwood Publishing Company, 1987.

Tracy, David. *How to Use Hypnosis*. New York: Sterling Publishing Company, 1952.

Van Pelt, S. J., M.D. *Secrets of Hypnotism*. Hollywood: Wilshire Book Company, 1976.

Wilson, Donald L., M.D. *Total Mind Power*. Los Angeles: Camero Publishing Co., 1976.

Weitzenhoffer, Andre. *Modern Hypnosis*. Hollywood: Wilshire Book Company, 1977.

Wyckoff, James. *Franz Anton Mesmer—Between God and Devil*. Englewood Cliffs: Prentice-Hall Inc., 1975.

Wynn, Ralph. *Hypnotism Made Easy*. Hollywood: Wilshire Book Company, 1978.

Young, L. E. *25 Lessons in Hypnotism*. New York: Padell Book Company, 1963.

Zeig, Jeffrey K. *Ericksonian Approaches to Hypnosis and Psychotherapy*. New York: Brunner/Mazel, Publishers, 1982.

Zeig, Jeffrey K. *Experiencing Erickson—An Introduction to the Man and His Work*. New York: Brunner/Mazel, Publishers, 1985.

Zilbergeld, Bernie, and Lazarus, Arnold A. *Mind Power: Getting What You Want Through Mental Training*. Toronto: Little, Brown and Company, 1987.

Index